A Practical Guide to Congenital Developmental Disorders and Learning Difficulties

To give children with congenital developmental conditions the best chance to succeed, early identification of their special learning needs and specific disabilities is necessary, as are the appropriate interventions and support.

This text highlights what to look for when there are concerns about a child's development. Practical and accessible, it is divided into three sections:

- Part 1 looks at the theory and policy context, discussing the social model of disability, the responsibility of health, social care and education services to the child and family and the role of reviews and assessment in recognizing developmental disorders.
- Part 2 provides a reference guide to atypical developmental conditions and disorders. For each condition, aetiology, prominent theories and research and profiles of features – including triggers and behaviours, diagnostic assessment procedures and appropriate interventions – are given and links made to sources of further information and support.
- Part 3 explores practical issues about how to work sensitively and effectively with children and their families, looking at the psychological implications of diagnosis, and how to plan, promote, deliver and evaluate multi-agency support.

Designed to support professionals working within a multi-modal, collaborative approach to assessment and intervention processes, this book is suitable for health visitors, allied health therapists, nurses, teachers and social care practitioners. It is also a useful reference for students in these areas learning about child development and includes critical reading exercises, online searching tasks, self-assessment questions, reflective activities and document analysis prompts.

Judith P. Hudson, PhD, is a former teacher, assessor and lecturer in special education needs and specific learning disorders at the University of Gloucestershire, UK, and is currently an Honorary Research Associate at the University of Tasmania, Australia.

With valuable guidance from **Sarah E. Henton**, BSc (Hons) SCPHN (HV), a qualified health visitor and experienced practice nurse working in rural Herefordshire, UK.

A Practical Guide to Congenital Developmental Disorders and Learning Difficulties

Judith P. Hudson

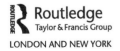

Routledge
Taylor & Francis Group

LONDON AND NEW YORK

First published 2014
by Routledge
2 Park Square, Milton Park, Abingdon, Oxon, OX14 4RN

and by Routledge
711 Third Avenue, New York, NY 10017

Routledge is an imprint of the Taylor & Francis Group, an informa business

© 2014 Judith P. Hudson

British Library Cataloguing in Publication Data
A catalogue record for this book is available from the British Library

Library of Congress Cataloging-in-Publication Data
Hudson, Judith P., author.
A practical guide to congenital developmental disorders and learning difficulties / Judith P. Hudson.
p. ; cm.
Includes bibliographical references.
Summary: "To give children with congenital developmental conditions that manifest special learning needs and specific disabilities their best chance to succeed, early identification and appropriate interventions and support, is necessary. This text highlights what to look for when there are concerns about a child's development. Practical and accessible, it is divided into three sections: - Part 1 looks at the theory and policy context, discussing the social model of disability, the responsibility of health, social care and education services to the child and family and the role of reviews and assessment in recognising developmental disorders. - Part 2 provides a reference guide to atypical developmental conditions and disorders. For each condition, aetiology, prominent theories and research, profile of features - including triggers and behaviours, diagnostic assessment procedures and appropriate interventions are given and links made to sources of further information and support. - Part 3 explores practical issues how to work sensitively and effectively with children and their families, looking at the psychological implications of diagnosis, and how to plan, promote, deliver and evaluate multi-agency support. Designed to support professionals working within a multi-modal, collaborative approach to assessment and intervention processes, it is suitable for health visitors, allied health therapists, nurses, teachers and social care practitioners. It is also a useful reference for students in these areas learning about child development and includes critical reading exercises; online searching tasks; self-assessment questions; reflective activities and document analysis prompts"--Provided by publisher.
I. Title.
[DNLM: 1. Developmental Disabilities--diagnosis. 2. Child Care--methods. 3. Child. 4. Learning Disorders--diagnosis. 5. Social Support. WS 350.6]
RC570
616.85'88--dc23
2013040344

ISBN: 978-0-415-63378-9 (hbk)
ISBN: 978-0-415-63379-6 (pbk)
ISBN: 978-0-203-09479-2 (ebk)

Typeset in Sabon by
GreenGate Publishing Services, Tonbridge, Kent

For Samuel, Caitlin, Toby and Roisin:
four very special people

Contents

Tables

Activities

Foreword

Children with disabilities can be defined in the eyes of others more by their disability than by being a child. Then there is a double whammy, because instead of a holistic approach to their particular life as a child, they are subject to piecemeal services. This practical guide aims to change this situation by bringing together many different aspects of working with children with disabilities.

Judith Hudson's book begins by charting one country's struggle (the UK) to change through legislation by setting up different systems to support working together. There is emphasis throughout the book on working together, on multi-disciplinary work, on partnership working and showing the way forward for working with children and families in this situation.

This is an ambitious book, both in scope and in intention. The book is wide ranging, from systems through disorders and stopping off at Piaget and Vygotsky on the way. The summaries of concepts are clear and concise and provide a good introduction for new practitioners and a reminder for more experienced workers.

Being written by an educator, there are features in the book to aid learning. Every chapter begins with learning outcomes and finishes with a summary of main points, while in between there are activities to help engagement with the text.

Judith Hudson has a clear thinking mind; the definitions of MRI and fMRI (yes, this book is wide ranging!) are the clearest I have seen. So this book does provide a practical guide to this field and will be very handy to refresh knowledge.

The book concludes with its goal, that: 'The core understanding is that those who are the frontline service providers have the skills, knowledge and motivation to do the best they can, for those with the greatest need.' This is a book that will assist practitioners in keeping the child and their family in the heart of services.

Dr Hazel Douglas, MBE
Consultant Clinical Psychologist and Child Psychotherapist and
Director of Solihull Approach, Heart of England NHS Foundation Trust, UK

Preface

The purpose of this guide is to provide accessible information about congenital neurological and cognitive developmental disorders for professionals who work with children in the disciplines of health, social work or education. A new impetus by policy makers that began during the 1990s has increased, and a 'joined-up' model across, and between, interdisciplinary services has been strengthened. A raft of recent government initiatives in England and countries that comprise the UK have set out the pathway for reforms, and moved to blur boundaries between service providers in health, education and social care. Rather than working in a compartmentalized system, early identification of pervasive 'within-child' developmental disorders, and prompt delivery of appropriate intervention, falls to professionals and providers that come together to form a multiple range of services. Written within the traditions of social science enquiry, this book examines evolving policy and practice in health care, social and education systems, to support and inform professionals who serve the needs of the community. It is within this context that I focus.

In a universal, needs-led service the primary professional has been viewed traditionally as the health visitor (HV), with fundamental responsibility being to search for health needs and identify many conditions, normally at the time of birth or shortly after. But the congenital, neurological and cognitive disorders described here manifest additional or different learning needs and specific disabilities that may only become apparent as the infant encounters socialization patterns and settings in the developmental environment (e.g. childcare/early years setting, nursery or primary education). It is the nature of such disorders, and the nurturing within systems of the developmental environment, that form the corpus of this book.

Disorders that are congenital carry pre-determined conditions that will impact on normal or typical development. A disorder that is congenital *and* developmental will be present from birth but also change over time throughout the development of the child. To give children with such conditions the best chance to succeed in life, early identification of problems is crucial. Fortunately advances in neuroscience and genetics are increasing our knowledge of early indicators and recognition of disorders, and professional training enables those who have primary care responsibilities to be more alert to factors in the child's immediate environment that make him/her vulnerable or 'at risk' of developing particular conditions.

In the UK, change is gathering apace and being effected across disciplines of health, social care and education. A paradigm shift to a model of integrated collaborative service delivery brings new responsibilities and demands. If we are to improve outcomes for children from early pregnancy, through early years of life, adolescence and beyond, joint commissioning and integrated children's services across general practice, health and community services are essential to support children and their families. The health professional is at the frontline interface between the service providers and caregivers, and has a primary role as the key professional in community-based services, with a shared commitment to promoting the welfare, health and well-being of children. HVs, school, community and general practitioner nurses are the professionals best placed in this process. Screening, early identification of developmental anomalies, preventive health care and monitoring the child through developmental reviews is in their domain. All need to know what markers to look for in ante/post-natal infant checks, and early years.

This book offers a practical guide to normal, or typical, development through to an anomalous spectrum of atypical disorders that result in an adverse developmental trajectory for the child. It is an authoritative, practical guide for providers of services in which the developing child is placed. It aims to support professionals across agencies and working within a collaborative approach to assessment and intervention. I have attempted to provide generic information points, and a guide to reference sources for multi-agency professionals, public health care practitioners, and social and community workers. Through signpost markers, it will enable you to locate further information, research evidence or pursue your own enquiry. Equally, it will serve the needs of those who work in childcare services, or in the domains of Child and Adolescent Mental Health Services (CAMHS). It could also support and appeal to professionals in the making of judgements, providing guidance and direction, for those who deliver services and support through children's centres: teachers of pupils with special educational needs (SEN) and/or the SEN-coordinator (SENCO) alike.

I aim to help clarify multi-disciplinary issues and provide a reference resource for students who are studying archetypical (normal) and atypical (uncharacteristic) neurological development at the level of under and/or postgraduate health, social care or education. For frontline practitioners, this book will support the recognition of high and low incidence developmental conditions, and highlight what to look for at both ante/post-natal infant screening checks, and in early years settings. This will usefully alert health care professionals to anomalous triggers, or behaviours, in the child at an early developmental stage.

The disorders I have presented are covered systematically and comprehensively and based on widely accepted criteria from authoritative sources (e.g. diagnostic manuals as described in Chapter 3). Recommended reading references that I give at the end of each section will give you access to supporting information, reference works and websites; in some disorders there is a cross-reference to UK published clinical guidance from the National Institute for Health and Care Excellence (NICE). This will create supporting links to further specific clinical information.

The universal children's rights movement has worked to promote and enshrine in national and international law, society's duty to recognize, and address, the child's needs, and it is my belief that if children are given the opportunity to say something, they frequently provide genuinely new insights and common sense opinions. As we have become increasingly committed in the UK to a model of advocacy and policy, which promotes the active participation of children in all matters that concern them, I have suggested practical ways in which professionals can access, and take into account, the views and perspectives of children. Child advocacy should not focus exclusively on protecting children; it should also be about understanding their views since children often have a different perspective of the treatments and services that are provided for them by adults. As Melton (1987) argues, there are inherent ethical risks because of the transfer of power, from the adult to the child, that inevitably has to take place.

Although framed within the UK system, I have tried to present broad, general information and practical advice on specific disorders. A child with intellectual, physical or sensory disabilities will display remarkably similar characteristics, ante/post-natal and require almost identical forms of effective intervention no matter where they are in the world. This supports my view that sharing good practical strategies will have both appeal and international relevance. Legal mandates, regulations, codes of practice and administrative procedures, however, are those that are relevant to England, while also aligned to countries that have different assemblies and lawmakers but within the UK. Where relevant, these will be alluded to in the book.

I have employed a theoretical model of the developmental environment that gives a contextual framework applicable to examination of structural systems across different countries and cultures worldwide. The reference materials in this book will be useful to student or practitioner alike. I hope you will find this guide a book to come back to again and again to support, and inform, your professional practice, or direct and aid you in your search for additional sources of information.

Acknowledgements

I would like to extend my thanks to all those who have generously given me their time, and provided me with valuable information about so many aspects of developmental disorders. I am grateful too for the acceptance of my presence in support groups in the UK, Australia and New Zealand. This involvement provides insights into the difficulties families experience when identification and support is not available, crucially in the child's early years. My admiration has no bounds for the extraordinary level of commitment that parents and families devote to their child, or children, with a developmental disorder, and no matter how complex a need.

My thanks also go to Jeni Wetton for her personal contribution, and to those who have been directly involved in the publishing of this text.

My sincere thanks go to my health advisor Sarah Henton to whom I am indebted for her enormous contribution throughout. Her informed guidance on all matters medical, health and care legislation, policies and structural systems within the universal health service has been invaluable. Sarah guided me through a labyrinth of information that, at the outset, appeared too daunting to ever comprehend. Without your inspiration and support, Sarah, this book really would not have happened.

Finally, my thanks to Duncan for his unwavering conviction in my abilities, his love and his support, and for never once counting the times I declared that the book was 'almost finished'.

How to use this book

For frontline practitioners, this book will support the recognition of high and low incidence developmental conditions, and highlight what to look for in ante/post-natal infant screening checks, and early years settings. This will usefully alert health care professionals to triggers, or adverse behaviours, in the child at an early developmental stage.

The book also has a practical and engaging dimension with design features to support easy access and understanding of the information you need to know. At the start of each chapter, keywords are given. Many are defined in the text, as are most of the acronyms, but others may be found in the glossary at the back of the book. This will ensure that the meaning of these words will become clear as you read through the chapter.

To support active learning and consolidate understanding of the concepts, contexts and themes, intended learning outcomes (ILO) are also given at the outset of each chapter. The structure of each chapter will integrate various self-teaching tasks and exercises that I propose as study aids. Guided answers to these questions can be found at the back of the book.

Activities include:

- Critical thinking to show that you understand the strengths and weaknesses, as well as the main idea of the work in question. Smith's (1995: 2) definition is applied here as 'logical and rational process of avoiding one's preconceptions by gathering evidence, contemplating and evaluating alternatives, and coming to a conclusion'.
- Using the Internet as a resource: online searching tasks to learn how to be selective, focused and discerning, and avoid becoming overwhelmed or frustrated by the enormous amount of information, and *mis*information, that is published on the Internet.
- Self-assessment questions (SAQs) to test your own knowledge or understanding.
- Developing reflective tasks: to consider your own practices and explore potential changes that can be made.

Finally, a summary of issues covered in each chapter is given. Directions to further reading and reference pathways are also provided to direct you to useful sources of information, including: the National Health Service (NHS); the National Institute for Health and Care Excellence (NICE) clinical guidelines; and leading UK charities for those with a specific disorder and their families (e.g. Williams Syndrome Foundation; the National Autistic Society (NAS); or Asperger's Syndrome Foundation (ASF)).

Abbreviations

AAC	augmentative and alternative communication
ABA	Applied Behavioural Analysis
ADHD	attention deficit hyperactivity disorder
APA	American Psychiatric Association
AS	Asperger Syndrome
ASD	autism spectrum disorder
ASF	Asperger Syndrome Foundation
CAF	Common Assessment Framework
CAMHS	Child and Adolescent Mental Health Service
CBT	Cognitive Behavioural Therapy
CNS	central nervous system
CP	cerebral palsy
CPD	continued professional development
CSF	cerebrospinal fluid
DAMP	Deficits in Attention, Motor Control and Perceptual Abilities
DCD	developmental coordination disorder
DD	developmental dyslexia
DDA	Disability Discrimination Act
DfE	Department for Education
DH	Department of Health
DNA	deoxyribonucleic acid
DSM	*Diagnostic and Statistical Manual of Mental Disorders*
DVD	Developmental Verbal Dyspraxia
ECM	Every Child Matters
EEG	electroencephalography
EHCP	Education Healthcare Plan
EYFS	Early Years Foundation Stage
FAS	Foetal Alcohol Syndrome
FASD	Foetal Alcohol Spectrum Disorder
fMRI	functional magnetic resonance imaging
FNP	Family Nurse Partnership
GFCF	gluten-free casein-free
GP	general practitioner
HCP	Healthy Child Programme
HFA	high-functioning autism
HGC	Human Genetics Commission

HV	health visitor
ICD	*International Statistical Classification of Diseases and Related Health Problems*
ICS	Integrated Children's System
IPSEA	Independent Parental Special Education Advice
IQ	intelligence quotient
LA	local authority
LoC	locus of control
LSCB	Local Safeguarding Children Board
MBD	minimal brain dysfunction
MRI	magnetic resonance imaging
NAS	National Autistic Society
NHS	National Health Service
NICE	National Institute for Health and Care Excellence
NMC	Nursing and Midwifery Council
NOFAS	National Organisation for Foetal Alcohol Syndrome
NSPCC	National Society for the Protection of Cruelty to Children
NT	neurotypical
OT	occupational therapy
PDD	pervasive developmental disorder
PDD-NOS	pervasive developmental disorder – not otherwise specified
PET	positron emission tomography
RS	Rett Syndrome
SA	Solihull Approach
SEAL	Social and Emotional Aspects of Learning
SEN	special educational needs
SENCO	SEN-coordinator
SENDA	Special Educational Needs and Disability Act
SGS	Schedule of Growing Skills
SL	speech and language
SLCN	speech, language and communication needs
SLT	speech and language therapist
SPD	Semantic Pragmatic Disorder
SpLD	Specific Learning Difficulties
SS	Sure Start
STD	sexually transmitted disease
TAC	team around the child
ToM	theory of mind
TR	text revision
UNCRC	United Nations Convention on the Rights of the Child
WBS	Williams-Beuren Syndrome (also Williams Syndrome (WS))
WHO	World Health Organization
WISC	Wechsler Intelligence for Children

Part 1

The dynamics of health, special education and disability in the UK

Chapter 1   **Effecting social change**

Intended learning outcomes

At the end of this chapter you will

- know and understand key statutory and regulatory frameworks and key developments in universal public health and associated education and care services in England;
- understand what philosophies underpin the *medical* and *social* models of disability;
- know the legal definition of *special educational needs* (SEN);
- understand how modelling a social framework can inform about extraneous influences that impact child health and development;
- be aware of the importance of accessing the child's perspective and considering the views of the child in any assessment programme;
- understand how safeguarding and child protection policy and practice are paramount in all services that deal with children and young people; and
- understand the importance and the value of professional ethical codes and essential guidelines.

Key words (defined in the text)

Bioecological, child protection, ecological systems, ethics, nature, nurture, reciprocity, safeguarding, social modelling.

Introduction

In this chapter, I shall first explore the dynamics of the current universal health service in England, and the countries that comprise the United Kingdom; universal services being services available to everyone. The sheer volume of political activity and involvement deems this first chapter heavily weighted towards how the process has been, and is being, implemented. I focus on relevant key legislation and non-statutory guidance from the plethora of politically motivated initiatives that continue to evolve in the first decades of the twenty-first century. These will address key reforms in health, special education, disability and social care from the final decades of the last century through to current 'evolving' systems. I have cited systems that have territorial extent in England and Wales, and that have shaped integrated working practices for multi-discipline professionals to effectively deliver frontline services. Next, I shall identify inherent factors that can be observed in the shaping of universal provision of health and well-being services. I describe legally defined models of disability and SEN, then present a favoured model for understanding forces within social systems, the impact of environmental factors on development and introduce the construct of reciprocity (Bronfenbrenner 1979). I shall present techniques through which to gain access to the voice and point of view of the child, or children's, perspective; safeguarding and child protection that essentially have to be addressed are also discussed. Finally, ethics and ethical codes of conduct and practice are introduced.

Historical perspectives – twenty-first-century key legislation: an overview

A range of legislation policies and services have accumulatively shifted the dynamics of delivered multi-agency early years health, education and social care service. The territorial extent and application of laws cited here apply to England and Wales, but with the majority only applying to England. Similar key statutes can also be found in Northern Ireland and Scotland and a self-teaching exercise in this chapter provides an opportunity to examine the systems model in each UK nation. These ongoing changes address priorities identified by managers, practitioners and experts from across local government, the National Health Service (NHS), social care and special education services. Since the beginning of the new millennium, policy makers have, in continuum, set out the pathway for ongoing reforms, including several models of provision that have been short-lived under shifting political influences. The concept of multi-agency involvement has also taken root in other countries where similar administration systems exist, for example Canada, New Zealand and Australia.

The first notable social intervention initiative highlighted is Sure Start (SS) in 1999, a programme introduced in the UK to tackle deprivation and embrace social inclusion, and is a prominent link in the changes I outline here. NHS policy, initiatives and a raft of politically motivated legislation established practice support tools such as an Integrated Children's System (ICS) and ContactPoint. Every Child Matters (ECM) (2003) aimed to get coordinated help quickly and through integrated services for children in need from 0–19 years; the Children Act (2004); the National Service Framework for children and young people and maternity services: Change for Children – Every Child Matters in 2004, a ten-year plan, and the Common Assessment Framework (CAF) (DfES 2009) moved the transition along towards a multi-agency model of service provision across professional boundaries. The ECM made a commitment to partnership and a multi-agency framework within the Children's Services proposals and was the precursor of the CAF. The CAF was developed through regional trials in England between 2005 and 2006, evaluated by the University of East Anglia and, when introduced to the wider population, this offered an applied conceptual framework for working with children in need and their families.

With the emergence of a coalition government in 2010, subtle policy changes evolved and, at a time of international and national economic crises, change was often necessary, and motivated, through reduced financial investment. However, the previous decade had introduced a generic and holistic way for all professionals to follow the same procedure, to gather and record information that consolidated the move towards collaboration across frontline services. It was designed to help practitioners assess needs at a developmentally early stage. The primary objective of both an ICS and the CAF was to provide coordinated professional help, particularly for children with additional needs and their families, and to focus on prevention and early intervention while providing better support to parents and families. Procedurally, it aimed at providing a more efficient use of information, systematically collected by professionals to improve the well-being and safeguarding of children at risk. The procedures within the CAF placed children and young people at the heart of the process. This centrality of the child in all matters concerning them was stimulated by the United Nations Convention on the Rights of the Child (UNCRC) (1989). Part 1, Article 12, states that:

> Parties shall assure to the child who is capable of forming his or her own views the right to express those views freely in all matters affecting the child, the views of the child being given due weight in accordance with the age and maturity of the child.
>
> (UNCRC 1989, Article 12)

Other substantive children's rights include the right to:

- special protection measures and assistance;
- access services such as education and health care;
- develop their personalities, abilities and talents to the fullest potential;
- grow up in an environment of happiness, love and understanding; and
- be informed about, and participate in, achieving their rights in an accessible and active manner.

The voice of the child must be heard and legislation is in place that makes explicit that the wishes and feelings of children are to be given due consideration in matters, or decisions, that concern them. Strategies for consulting children or eliciting the child's perspective are first introduced later in this chapter and link to themes in this book that include: ethics and safeguarding (Chapter 1), child development and developmental surveillance (Chapter 2); placing the child central to the assessment (Chapter 3); processes in making a diagnosis (Chapters 4 and 5); gaining the perspective of the child with a disorder and psychosocial issues that are a secondary consequence of living with a developmental disorder (Chapter 6); listening and hearing the voices of children (Chapter 7); and working with the parents (Chapter 8). In conclusion, I bring it all together to look at 'the way forward' (Chapter 9).

To further improve desired outcomes for all children and young people, policies extending from ECM and CAF include: Youth Matters in 2005, the Children's Plan in 2007 and the 2020 Children and Young People's Workforce Strategy in 2008 aimed at promoting priority outcomes given by the ECM and summarized in Table 1.1. In 2007, the Family Nurse Partnership (FNP) programme for young first time mothers was rolled out, and was funded in areas of England with high social and economic deprivation. This initiative, first established in the US as the Nurse Family Partnership (NFP) before being introduced in England, had three fundamental aims: to improve pregnancy outcomes by helping women to improve pre-natal health; to improve child health and development by helping parents provide sensitive and competent care of the child; and to improve the course of parental life by helping parents plan future pregnancies, complete their education and to find work to improve parents' economic self-sufficiency. The programme provides a schedule of intensively structured home visiting by specially trained nurses, from early pregnancy until the child's second birthday, and the initiative is underpinned by theories of human ecology, self-efficacy and attachment.

TABLE **1.1** Every Child Matters (ECM) outcomes and aims bringing multi-agency support services together to support children and young people through the CAF

	Outcomes	*Aims*
Be healthy	Physically healthy Mentally and emotionally healthy Sexually healthy	Healthy lifestyles Choose not to take illegal drugs
Stay safe	Safe from maltreatment, neglect, violence and exploitation Safe from accidental injury and death Safe from bullying and discrimination	Safe from crime and antisocial behaviour in and out of school Have security, stability and cared for
Enjoy and achieve	Ready for school Attend and enjoy school Achieve stretching national educational standards at primary school	Achieve personal and social development, and enjoy recreation Achieve stretching national educational standards at secondary school
Make a positive contribution	Engage in decision-making and support the community and environment Engage in law abiding and positive behaviour in and out of school	Develop positive relationships; choose not to bully and discriminate Develop self-confidence and successfully deal with significant life changes and challenges Develop enterprising behaviour
Achieve economic well-being	Engage in further education, employment or training on leaving school Ready for employment Live in decent homes and sustainable communities	Access to transport and material goods Live in households free from poverty

Guidance from the Department of Health (DH) came in the Healthy Child Programme (HCP) and concerned the delivery of services to children from 0–5 years (DH 2009). It set out universal preventive services for families, and focused on screening, immunization, health and development reviews, and health and well-being. It emphasized parent support and looked to engage fathers and was extended through Supporting Children and Young People's Health: from 5–19 Years Old, in 2010. This aimed to build on developing further the universal and progressive framework of support for children and young people. It also outlined responsibilities for local commissioners of services, health, education and social care and other partners to deliver integrated services at the local level. In the process of transforming community-based services Healthy Lives, Healthy People: Our Strategy for Public Health in England (2010) proposed five phases of a life course given as: Starting Well, Developing Well, Living Well, Working Well, and Aging Well that underpin a key framework. Reforming the public health system in England continued with the Health Visitor Implementation Plan (July–September 2012) that expanded and strengthened the health visiting services and was pivotal to the extension of initiatives cited here. This involved recruitment and training of a further 4,200 HVs across England essential to successfully implement local, high-quality programmes.

Another key player recognized as 'crucial' in the lead and delivery of the HCP and strengthening a 'rejuvenated workforce' (DH 2012) is the school nurse. This specialist public health nurse works with the school-age population (5–19 years) to assess health and well-being needs, and can lead and influence health promotion activities both in, and out of, the school setting. Qualified school nurses are graduate level professionals, the qualification of which leads to registration as a Specialist Community Public Health Nurse (SCPHN). The emphasis in their role is on identification, preventive and promotion of health and well-being. The school nurse in England works in collaboration with key professionals in health, social care and SEN. In areas of high social need, the service complements and supports the FNP to integrate provision within universal health, education and social services. Applying evidence from neuroscience to inform practice in supporting children and young people, other issues that school nurses cover include:

- supporting early intervention in mental ill health, and identifying and helping children and young people, and their families, who need support with their emotional or mental health;
- monitoring excess weight in 4–5 and 10–11-year-olds;
- promoting emotional well-being of looked after children;
- reducing smoking prevalence in 15-year-olds;
- reducing alcohol and drug misuse;
- reducing under 18 conception rates; and
- monitoring tooth decay in five-year-olds.

Key statutes, guidance and public health initiatives central to the shaping of twenty-first-century child health care in England are summarized below.

1999   Sure Start (SS) programme, the first integrated early years services
1989, 2004 Children Act
2002–2003   Every Child Matters: Change for Children

2004–2014	Healthy Child Programme 0–5 (DH 2009); National Service Framework (NSF) for children, young people and maternity services (DH 2004)
2007	Family Nurse Partnership (FNP)
2009	Common Assessment Framework (CAF) (DfES 2009)
2009	Healthy Child Programme (HCP) (DH 2009)
2010	Healthy Lives, Healthy People
2011–2015	Reformed strategy for public health in England: Health Visitor Implementation Plan (July–September 2012)
2011–2012	Health Visitor One Year On
2012	Health and Social Care Act
2012	Statutory Framework for Early Years Foundation Stage (EYFS)
2013	Children and Families Bill.

The document Health Visitor One Year On in 2011–2012 reported changes being realized at a local level, and within the shared assessment and planning framework the strategy for Children and Young People's Health (DH 2009) had proposed. The development of an integrated service model has translated to practice, broadly delineated through the corpus of guidance and legislation reported here. Overlapping health and social care legislation and support continues to develop an integrated, multi-disciplinary service, evident in England's contemporary support systems. The statutory framework for the EYFS (DfE 2012a: 2) sets out standards that early years service providers have to meet to 'ensure that children learn and develop well and are kept safe'. Moving further towards multi-agency collaboration, partnership is advocated between practitioners, carers and parents. The need for an enabling environment that covers the education and care of all children in early years provision, including children with SEN and/or disability, is advocated. It also makes clear the duty for practitioners to consider whether a child may have a special educational need or disability that requires specialist support that links with, and helps families to access, relevant services from other agencies as appropriate. How special education and social care structures have evolved towards an integrated model of provision is described in the summary below. Key legislation and statutory guidance codes are also highlighted.

Activity 1.1: Internet and online search

Since 2000, Scotland, Northern Ireland and Wales, as well as England, have each developed their own changes in practice and moved towards integrated models of provision. What were the relevant Acts and resultant initiatives that directed change in the three other countries that comprise the UK?

Terminology: special educational needs and models of disability

First coined by the Warnock Report, the term 'special educational needs' appeared in the report from an enquiry, guided by Mary Warnock (later Baroness Warnock), into the education of 'handicapped children and young people' (Warnock 1978). This significant and comprehensive report summarized findings from a survey as to what provision was available for children with physical and intellectual difficulties in the UK in the late 1970s. From this came the 1981 Education Act that radically changed the nature of education policy and philosophy not just in the UK but internationally. It set out the collective responsibilities to identify, provide for and support children assessed as having a learning difficulty or a SEN. The most significant change in philosophy was from a bias towards segregated provision, or placing children in special schools according to their 'handicap' or disability, and instead to develop inclusive practices. Here *all* children had the right to an education in an ordinary or mainstream school. So too was negative language such as 'retarded', 'subnormal' or 'handicapped' abandoned. Over time legislation, regulations, codes of conduct and political initiatives, aligned predominantly to the international 'rights' movement, have changed the education experience of those children with a developmental disorder. The Warnock Report concluded that 20 per cent of children in the school population could have a SEN but 2 per cent might need support over, and above, what a mainstream school could provide for.

The 1988 Education Act made legal a demand for all schools to provide a national curriculum and thus allow access to equal education for *all* children. This notably was the first commitment to equality in education regardless of ability or disability in the UK. In the 1990s change accelerated, starting in 1994 for education of children with a SEN when two major events made an impact. First, June 1994 saw the issue of the United Nations Educational Scientific and Cultural Organization (UNESCO 1994) Salamanca (Spain) Statement. Article 24 reinforced the notion and commitment to inclusive education for all pupils, unless there were compelling reasons for doing otherwise. The UK became signatories and ratified this statement along with 92 governments and 25 non-governmental organizations (NGOs); only two countries did not ratify (Somalia and the United States). Thus international agreement made a dynamic statement about the education of all disabled children, and made inclusion into an ordinary or mainstream school the norm.

That year also saw the introduction of a SEN Code of Practice in England and Wales (DfES 1994) which laid down a process of five stages that education professionals and local authorities were *advised* to follow, or to which schools were to 'have a regard'. Stages one to four provided support through the school, then external specialist services, and Stage five was the stage whereby a 'Statement of SEN' could be written, a legally binding document that the local authority (LA) had to abide by, and specifying exact provision over and above other children of the same age. Amended in 2002, a new system was introduced: School Action and School Action Plus, and Early Years Action and Early Years Action Plus for all early years educational settings. This was the new process through which to identify SEN, and the 'statement' system for those with more severe and/or complex needs continued. Four broad areas, within which developmental disorders are grouped, form the SEN spectrum: communication and interaction; cognition and learning; behaviour, emotional and social development; and sensory and physical needs. The disorders described in Chapters 4 and 5 will rarely fit into these clear-cut categories and often overlap. For example, disorders on the autism spectrum impact on communication and interaction, cognition and learning *and* domains such as social and emotional development and sensory experiences. The presence of more than one condition, or co-morbidity, also leads to an overlap as becomes apparent in later chapters.

Part 2 of the Special Educational Needs and Disability Act (SENDA) (2001) was reflected in the SEN Code of Practice (DfES 2002). The Act was then modified and became Part 4 of the Disability Discrimination Act (DDA) (1995), which was itself amended later (2005). This placed a duty to provide equal opportunity to all disabled people, and aimed to ensure that all young persons achieve full potential. Where possible, this was to be within a mainstream school and it made explicit that schools were prohibited from discriminating against disabled children in their admissions arrangements, and in the education and associated services provided by schools for its pupils.

A plethora of government legislation on disability and special education have passed through political systems in the past three decades, far too numerous to detail here, but the most significant and influential reports, statutes, initiatives and guidance in the development of support for children with SEN and/or disabilities are given below. The core reports, reviews and most influential legislation are also summarized below.

1978	Warnock Report on specialist provision and support for pupils with SEN
1981	Education Act: responsibility for SEN support passed to LEA
1988	Education Act – national curriculum for *all* children
1993	Education Act – reinforced/surpassed the 1981 Act
1994	Code of Practice for SEN guidance – five stages and SEN 'Statements'
1996	Education Act – consolidated 1993 Act. Securing special education provision
1997	Excellence for all children – meeting SEN guidance
1998	From exclusion to inclusion – guidance
2001	SEN and Disability Act (SENDIS) – amended the 1996 Act
2002	Code of Practice for SEN, revised edition – reinforced SENDIS Act
2003	Every Child Matters – commitment to multi-agency partnerships
2004	Children Act – built on and extended 1989 Children Act
2008	Early Years Foundation Stage (EYFS) – 'standards' for childcare
2013	Children and Families Bill – reforms the SEN system.

The Children and Families Bill (2013) is briefly mentioned below but I return to it in more detail in later chapters (see Chapter 9). The Bill delivers the legislative commitments made in the Green Paper Support and Aspiration: A New Approach to Special Educational Needs and Disability: Progress and Next Steps (DfE 2012a) and was informed by reviews and reports such as:

- The SEN and disability review: a statement is not enough (Ofsted 2010).
- The Lamb enquiry – SEN and parent confidence (Lamb 2009).
- Better communication: a review of services for children and young people with speech, language and communication needs (SLCN) (Bercow 2008).
- Identifying and Teaching Children and Young People with Dyslexia and Literacy Difficulties (Rose 2009).
- The Salt Review – independent review of teacher supply for pupils with severe, profound and multiple learning difficulties (Salt 2010).

In England, Part 3 of the Children and Families Bill (2013) states that: 'A child or young person has SEN if he or she has a learning difficulty or disability which calls for special educational provision to be made for him or her' (10 (1), lines 25–27) and adds that:

A child of compulsory school age or a young person has a learning difficulty or disability if he or she:
  (a) has a significantly greater difficulty in learning than the majority of others of the same age; or
  (b) has a disability which prevents or hinders him or her from making use of facilities of a kind generally provided for others of the same age in mainstream schools or mainstream post-16 institutions.

((2), lines 28–34)

(Reproduced under the terms of Open Parliament Licence from the Draft Children and Families Bill (Bill 168), 25 April 2013)

Models of disability are well documented and enshrined in national law aligned to international decrees. The two most frequently used models in the UK are the *medical model* and *social model* of disability. The *medical* model views disability as a problem that is placed within the individual. It is seen as an issue that belongs to those with impairments, and defines disabled people by their illness or condition, depicts disabled persons as dependent and in need of being cured, or cared for, and, it could be argued, gives justification as to how those with a disability have been systematically excluded in society.

Disabled people worldwide have challenged this over-medicalization account of disability (Shakespeare 2006: 197) and instead 'the disability movement focused onto social oppression, cultural discourse and environmental barriers'. More recently there has been a paradigm shift, reflected in UK policy and practice, moving towards a social understanding of disability. The social model sees the problem as being a shared responsibility that collectively a society has a part in overcoming and draws on the idea that it is society that disables people. Disability then is viewed not as the fault of the disabled person, or an inevitable consequence of their limitations. A social model takes account of disabled people as part of the economic, environmental and cultural society. The duty is on society to legally remove discrimination and, by removing attitudinal, physical and financial barriers that governments have a moral duty to do, make an environment accessible to all. This 'moral duty' is enshrined in the international human rights instrument the United Nations Convention on the Rights of Persons with Disabilities (UNCRPD), ratified by the UK in 2009. Systems and access that are barriers to those with a disability have to be modified to enable access to all members of society regardless. This model underpins current policy and practice in the UK. The amended DDA (2005) was repealed, and replaced, by the Equality Act (HM Government 2010b), a UK civil rights law that makes it unlawful to discriminate against disabled people. It also requires service providers to make 'reasonable adjustments' in relation to the physical features of their premises.

Legislation that targeted discriminatory attitudes and behaviour towards those disadvantaged, physically or intellectually, through disability or impairment, is summarized in Table 1.2. These include international laws that strengthened earlier laws laid down in the UK, especially the Equality Act 2010. This consolidates the protected characteristics of disability as defined in earlier laws and prohibits discrimination through a range of circumstances, provision of goods, facilities and services, the exercise of public functions, premises, work, education and associations (HM Government 2010b).

TABLE 1.2 Summarized key disability, child welfare/safeguarding and social care legislation and initiatives

Year	Title	Core concepts
1989, 2005	Children Act	Welfare of child paramount Protection from harm Improve the lives of children
1999	Protection of Children Act	Identify those 'not suitable' to work with children
2001	The Special Educational Needs and Disability Act (SENDIS)	Amended the Disability Discrimination Act (1995) Unlawful to discriminate against disabled pupils Responsibility to make reasonable adjustments so disabled pupils not disadvantaged
2002	Education Act (Section 175)	Schools/local authorities 'safeguarding' responsibilities
2003 (DfES)	Laming Report: keeping children safe	Looked at need to change laws of child protection
2004	Children Act	Children's Commissioner for England LA elect lead member for children's service Local Safeguarding Children Boards given statutory duties
2004	Sir Michael Bichard Inquiry	Introduced centralized 'vetting' procedures
2008	The Children and Young Person Act	Transform the lives of children in care Ensure high-quality care and support
2010	Equality Act	Consolidated numerous Acts and Regulations Clarifies duty to 'remove barriers'
2011	Munro Review of Child Protection: final report	Need for a more child-focused system Reduction in prescriptive targets and timescales
April 2012 (DfE)	Revised Statutory Guidance	Response to findings in Munro Review Guidance for all professionals that work with children

The main elements of the definition of disability are given as:

A1 A person has a disability for the purposes of the Act if he or she has a physical or mental impairment and the impairment has a substantial and long-term adverse effect on his or her ability to carry out normal day-to-day activities (S 6 (1)).

A2 This means that, in general:
  • the person must have an impairment that is physical or mental (see **paragraphs A3 to A8**);
  • the impairment must have adverse effects which are substantial (see **Section B**);
  • the substantial adverse effects must be long-term (see **Section C**); and
  • the long-term substantial adverse effects must be effects on normal day-to-day activities (see **Section D**).

(HM Government 2010b, Equality Act 2010 Guidance)

This concludes the clarification of terms, and I end with a definition of what a congenital, or present since birth, developmental disorder is. A broad description is any condition that appears early on in a child's life and delays or impedes normal or expected patterns of development. It can be domain specific, e.g. characterized as affecting psychological, cognitive or physical development, and/or may also involve sensory or motor skill development. For salience, a pervasive developmental disorder (PDD) is characterized by a serious distortion of basic psychological functioning and may involve social, cognitive, perceptual, attention, motor or linguistic functioning (Reber and Reber 2001). Being developmental it will also change over time, particularly as the child reaches puberty and eventual maturation.

There is generally assumed to be no cure, but interventions can slow down and may reduce negative consequences of a disorder. Learning issues can be addressed through intervention, so as to reduce, or circumvent, resultant affective social, behavioural and/or cognitive learning difficulties. Labels are profuse, and often confusing, and terminology can be specific, or provide a broad frame of reference within which the disorder can best be understood. From a socio-constructivist perspective, disabilities can be understood partially in terms of social constructs and the term 'developmental disorder' viewed as a confusing mix of scientific theory, political advocacy and convenience for the delivery of services. Logically then it may seem, the wider the net is cast by terminology and labels, the more vague the terms become. What should have become apparent through this examination of description and definition is the inconstancy of constructs and the fluid dynamics of definition and labels over time. Change is usually in response to prevailing conditions at any given time, in any community, and this can be socially, politically or economically motivated, if not induced by all three variables.

There follows an overview of an ecological model of the developmental environment, a social model through which variables are contextualized that have gone some way towards influencing dynamics within systems discussed above.

Social modelling: ecological systems theory

In child development, both biological and environmental factors exert their respective influences and a key issue is where the different emphasis on their importance is placed. Health outcomes too are multi-determined and the result of complex interactions of many factors over time. The fundamental contributions that impact though stem from the child's biology and ecology. In psychology, this debate is more commonly described as the nature–nurture debate.

Nature includes genetic factors and biological influences during the period from conception through infancy, childhood, adolescence and beyond. It includes effects of disease and congenital, physical or psychological developmental disorders. Nurture includes influences in the developmental environment from family, community and the immediate cultural environment, and includes the influence of the wider society within which the developing child is placed. Contributions from research over the past decade, including the sequencing of the human genome, have moved science beyond the single agents of health, developmental conditions and disease to a broader systems perspective, based on the understanding that health outcomes result from multiple determinants and their interactions (Evans and Stoddart 1990).

Taking account of human factors can provide useful, important information, but factors operating in the social systems of the developmental environment also need to be considered. Developmental science and public policy makers require a methodologically substantial paradigm and here I present one such theoretical model. Through this examination of such factors within the child's developmental ecology becomes possible, and I try to elicit features inherent in social systems to then consider how these can interact with, and impact on, human factors. Through this, the recognition of wide ranging developmental influences can become possible as it allows for them to be observed.

In the field of developmental psychology, such a model allows for identification of interacting variables both within the individual, and the ecology wherein the individual is raised. It is favoured here because it offers a theoretical, operational and universal approach for investigating the role of the environment in shaping human development through the life course of the individual. It takes account of changing and consistent practices, beliefs and values within any culture or society. It may not allow for generalizations to be made, but I do consider it a tool robust enough through which to conduct research and/or to transfer enquiry as a framework to identify inherent systems in demographically different populations.

It is placed within both social interaction and cultural mediation theory, and derived from the traditions of Vygotsky (1962) whose philosophy of human development I discuss further in the next chapter. Bronfenbrenner's (1979) ecology of human development and socialization model introduced here, fundamentally underpinned the design and implementation of health, social and educational reforms such as the SS programme in the UK derived from the earlier Head Start programme in the US. Connections are made and contextualized within a paradigm that Bronfenbrenner (1979: 21–22) posits involves

> the scientific study of the progressive, mutual accommodation, between an active, growing human being and the changing properties of the immediate settings in which the developing person lives, as this process is affected by relations between these settings, and by the larger contexts in which the setting are embedded.

A 'setting' is described as a place 'where people readily engage in face-to-face interaction' (Bronfenbrenner 1979: 22), for example the home, childcare, pre-school, school or playground. 'Development' Bronfenbrenner (1979: 3) defines as 'a lasting change in the way a person perceives and deals with his/her environment'.

Three features underpin his model of development: first, the developing child is viewed as a growing dynamic entity, not merely a 'tabula rasa on which the environment makes an impact' (ibid.: 21). Second, influence is bidirectional: the environment exerts an influence on the child, but requires a process of mutual accommodation, a two-directional interaction between the child and its environment, characterized by the concept of reciprocity. From the developmentalist stance, reciprocity is identified as a critical component in normal human development towards maturity. Third, the environment described as relevant to the developmental processes is not restricted to a single immediate setting but is extended and interconnected between other settings as well as to external influences from the wider and larger surroundings.

In social psychology, the interactions between the child and the systems within which they are placed, reciprocity is considered a strong determinant factor of human behaviour. It works at many different levels. First, from the basic mother/child two-person, or dyadic, relationship to its broader context where it can be viewed as a form of social obligation that can help to develop, and continue, positive relationships with people. The analogy made by Bronfenbrenner (1979) is that reciprocity is like a game of 'ping-pong' in which there is mutual feedback that produces progressively more complex patterns of interaction. The outcome of such mutual interactivity and inter-dependence between developing persons is that 'it produces its most powerful effects' (ibid.: 57).

Expanded, with the addition of the *chrono*system, a third dimension that encom-passes 'change or consistency over time not only in the characteristics of the person but also of the environment in which the person lives' (Bronfenbrenner 1994: 40). Bioecological systems theory provides a provocative framework for the study of chil-dren with disorders or disabilities through the stress it lays on the quality and context of the child's surroundings.

A particularly useful concept within the framework are 'social addresses', demo-graphic and socio-economic constructs, that allow enquiry to take account of multifarious factors present in the child's home and family environment. Factors such as family size and structure, marital status/age of parents/parents'/mother's educa-tion and profession or occupation, ordinal position of the child in the family, rural/urban location type, nationality and ethnicity, father's role in the family unit, absent/present fathers, social status and roles within the community, even personal attributes such as self-efficacy and parents' self-efficacy can all be considered through such a framework.

Bronfenbrenner (1989/1992) posits that such addresses take account of factors such as 'one vs. two parent families, home reared/home-care vs. day childcare, child in private school vs. public school; mother's employment status, how many times re-married' (ibid.: 193) and if the child's birth parents are married to each other. The concept of 'social addresses' can be used to categorize wider demographic and social constructs to look beyond what Bronfenbrenner (1989/1992) terms the 'environmen-tal label'. The concept allows for attention to be given to the people who are living with, and around, the developing child; asks what they are doing and how his or her activities and the action of others, and/or significant others, affect and interact with the child.

This dynamic model, that has over time undergone complex reforms, fundamen-tally conceives the ecological environment as an interconnectedness of systems, not linear, rather it sees influences constantly pass in, out, back, forth and across differ-ent systems nested in an arrangement of concentric structures, each within the next. Hypothesized then as having bidirectionality, it can operate at the level of behavioural genetics or interactions between different social influences.

Working out from the innermost level is the immediate setting containing the devel-oping child (the *micro*system), the genetic behavioural environment with influences from the nuclear single setting. Looking beyond the single settings to a second level (the *meso*system), relations and interconnections between the systems can be observed through interactional settings such as the extended family, pre- and post-natal services and early years learning settings. These, Bronfenbrenner suggests, can be as decisive for development as events taking place within a given setting, and are crucial when examining the relationship between the developing individuals and systems in their developmental environment.

At a third level (the *exo*system), the wider social environments that do not include children, but will affect them, are brought to account, for example the workplace of the parent(s) and social processes such as maternity or paternity leave, cultural child-rearing practices or any positive or negative change in the circumstances of the family. The overarching system (the *macro*system) incorporates bodies of knowledge, material resources and belief systems, whether political, spiritual or economic, and influences the processes, opportunity and life course options between, to and from all individuals and across each of the system structures. Thus traditions, institutional policies and laws that affect social care, health and educational opportunity are determined through these systems and also by the available resources of the culture.

Adding the further dimension (the *chrono*system) takes account of changes over the life course in family structure, such as socio-economic status, employment, place and location of residence and/or time management and achieving the right work/life balance, between home, family child rearing and time for building and sustaining family relationships (Bronfenbrenner 1994). The features of each ecological system are summarized in Table 1.3.

TABLE 1.3 Features of Bronfenbrenner's (1979, 1989/1992) ecological and bioecological (1994) systems theory

System	Area of influence
*Micro*system	A pattern of activities, roles and interpersonal relations experienced by the developing child in a given setting with particular physical and material characteristics. Immediate behavioural, genetic, environmental, biological influences that directly shape or affect manifested behaviour of the child.
*Meso*system	The interrelations among two or more settings in which the developing child actively participates, such as the relations between home and school, home/health care services, neighbourhood peer group, etc. Extending out through family and community influences. Family relationships, school relationships, peers and significant others that affect the development of the child's attitudes, expectations, etc.
*Exo*system	One or more settings that do not involve the developing person as an active participant, but in which events occur that affect, or are affected by, what happens in the setting containing the developing person. For example, workplace of the parent(s), maternity leave, childcare systems, school or class attended by a sibling, parents' network of friends, school governors, local education authority, etc.
*Macro*system	Consistencies in the form and content of the three lower-order systems (micro, meso, exo) or ideology underlying such consistencies. The laws of society, cultural values, resources of the culture that the child develops within, customs and attitudes.
*Chrono*system (1994)	The changes that occur over time, in family, community and systems. Allows also for examination of changes and differences across two or more time frames. For example, childhood in the UK in 1950 compared to childhood in 2010.

Bronfenbrenner's hypothesis sees no event as viewed in isolation, detached or removed from the living, developing and learning situation. On another level, his model sees that a child's development is profoundly affected by events that occur in settings in which he or she may not even be present, as well as by social and economic forces that interact environmentally.

Placing such procedures as the CAF, ICS or ECM within Bronfenbrenner's (1979, 1989/1992, 1994) model(s), it is possible to view processes and prevailing conditions that govern the course of the child's development in his/her own environment. A child's socio-cultural context will affect how he or she constructs reality and viewing the child's life context through the 'ecological systems' model allows for the layers of socio-cultural influence on the child's experiences of life, health care and education experience to be examined. Utilizing the model at the individual level allows for attitudes, social and economic factors to be teased out, and separated from within child issues or specific cognitive difficulties attributed to his or her developmental condition. The common structures for recording evidence-based information about a child, or young person, as laid down in the ECM and CAF, for example, covers three domains: the developmental needs of the child; parental capacity; and family and environmental factors. It is within the child's immediate environment or the *micro*system that proximal processes operate upon these domains.

It is also possible to identify conditions prevailing in, and across, the *meso*ytem wherein the child and the family are placed. It allows for professionals to take account of the social addresses around the child, the family's relationship with the wider community *and* their relationship between social services and other supporting agencies. Programmes such as SS and FNP essentially involve professionals working closely with children, and their families in need, in a supportive role not an authoritarian or judgemental capacity. Understanding the values and culture of the family, respecting them and building relationships can only contribute positively towards favourable outcomes. Policies and laws are all a part of the *macro*system and professionals too have to work within the parameters this system presents.

Framed within the *exo*system, account can be taken of settings wherein events occur that affect the child but wherein the child may not be directly present (e.g. parents' workplace, LA organization of services in the child's environment) or even occurred before the child was born (e.g. parent's marital status, stability in extended family relationships, mother's education, etc.).

Legal and social systems are a device through which to introduce accountability and guidance for professionals. ECM sets out a national framework with five stated key outcomes to well-being in childhood, shown in summary in Table 1.1. These aims are fundamental in guidance to help the child achieve and fulfil their potential, regardless of limiting or debilitating factors. Notably though, a change of political leadership influenced a priorities shift in the *macro*system in the UK when the 2010 government change impacted subtly on both the nature and resource investment in the ECM initiative. I return to this model again elsewhere throughout these chapters, and its usefulness will become apparent as, and when, complex issues and professional tensions are examined.

Activity 1.2: Developing reflective practices

a   What information about development will the ecological systems approach add to your understanding of pre-birth (0) to early years (age five) from the perspective of developmental psychology?

b   Using the framework of the ecological systems model of the developmental environment (Bronfenbrenner 1989/1992), identify one key initiative in England in the past decade, and resulting systemic influence within each system below, that you would consider as a variable that has impacted on i) the child; ii) the family; and iii) the community.

i) *micro*   ii) *meso*   iii) *exo*   iv) *macro*   v) *chronosystem*

c   The framework of this model of human development supports psychosocial and cultural enquiry to identify and examine social, political, economical, cultural, emotional and familial influences in the developmental environment. Thinking about two or three examples of child health issues that you have encountered, how useful would this model be to your own understanding of constraints, or opportunities, to affect changes *for your client or their family*?

Safeguarding, child protection and ethical issues

In every organization and every walk of life, in health, education and social care where children are central to their professional care and duty, those employed with children have a duty to show beyond reasonable doubt that they are aware of child protection issues and, as a professional working with children, the safeguarding steps that must be taken. Professionals also need to be aware of the vulnerable position they are placed in and for their own protection be fully informed. Policies clearly direct all agencies and should work to prevent children suffering harm, strive to promote sound child welfare, provide them with the services they require to address their identified needs and safeguard those children who are being, or who are likely to be, harmed.

Safeguarding practices are broader than 'child protection' and also include stringent preventative measures, yet although introduced after high-profile, child abuse fatalities such as those of Victoria Climbié (February 2000) and later baby Peter (August 2007), statistics still show that in the UK between 2007 and 2008 some 55 children were killed by a parent or by someone known to the child (Laming Report 2003). Such events continue to occur as exemplified by the death in 2012 of Daniel Pelka age four years, from starvation and untreated head injuries.

Further strategic change though has aimed to fundamentally improve UK child protection standards. Reforms introducing ever tighter safeguarding policies, legislation, structured guidance and procedures in England and UK countries continue to be formulated, aiming to avoid the recurrence of such tragic events or dire statistics. The Laming Report (2003) stipulated that strategic priorities for the protection of children and young people must be overt and fully integrated across key frontline services and, in response, a National Safeguarding Delivery Unit was established, was fully operational by July 2009 but abolished in 2012 when policy change followed a government change.

I have outlined policy that places a duty on those employed in multi-agency community services to keep children safe, and international laws that acknowledge all children have the right to be free from maltreatment or abuse. Professionals have a duty also to identify the children and families most in need and help them as early as possible. Health, special education and social care professionals must work together to prevent impairment to health or development, and ensure wherever possible all children in their care grow up in circumstances consistent with the provision of safe and effective care.

The Munro review of child protection (Munro 2011) strongly advocates collaboration that should aim to foster effective partnerships, provide effective protection and help children who are suffering, or likely to suffer, significant harm. Agencies such as the Royal College of Paediatrics and Child Health, the Royal College of General Practitioners, DH, the Department for Education (DfE) and local authorities should work together. International rulings (e.g. the 1996 Hague Convention; Safeguarding Vulnerable Groups (Northern Ireland) Order 2007 Schedule 2, Paragraph 5A) and the UK government response to the Munro review of child protection (2011) deemed that responsibility *must* be a joint venture.

Child protection should transcend central government, local agencies, local authorities and professionals. In England, the established Local Safeguarding Children Boards (LSCBs) have local statutory responsibility as a key mechanism for pulling together child protection measures, and plays a central role in keeping children and young people safe. Additionally, reforms to safeguarding shifted the focus of the child protection system on to what matters most, the views and experiences of children and young people, and places the emphasis on the voice of the child. Strategies that focus on accessing the child's perspective, the ethical issues and obligations are discussed later in this chapter and again in Chapter 7.

Children and young people with disabilities or special needs are around three times more likely to be abused or neglected, and are more likely to be at risk of abuse or neglect than non-disabled children. Safeguarding is therefore a major issue for such children and young people. There is also an entitlement to 'staying safe' in the five key areas of the ECM agenda (see Table 1.1). For frontline professionals, the National Society for the Protection of Cruelty to Children (NSPCC) is a UK organization that specializes in child protection, prevention of cruelty and abuse to children, and is signposted here as a route to a plethora of material and advice about safeguarding practice and/or legal responsibilities for children and professionals who work with them.

Key legislation

- UNCRC (1989)
- The Safeguarding Vulnerable Groups Act (2006)
- The Children Act (1989, 2004)
- The Human Rights Act (1998)

Relevant articles in the UNCRC

- **Articles 2, 3, 6 and 12** focus on non-discrimination, call for the best interests of the child, the right to life, survival and development and respect for the child's views.

- **Articles 5, 9, 10, 11, 18, 20, 21, 25** and **27** focus on care within or outside the family: covers issues such as parental responsibility, reviews of placements outside of the family, adoption.
- **Articles 18, 23, 24** and **27** focus on welfare and health: welfare issues, childcare services, standards of living and provision for disabled children.
- **Article 19** focuses on the right to protection from all forms of violence and injury, abuse, neglect or exploitation.
- **Article 23** focuses on the right of disabled children to special care, education and training to ensure the fullest possible social integration.

UK government guidance

- Working together to safeguard children: a guide to interagency to safeguard and promote the welfare of children (HM Government 2006).
- Mental health in children and young people: an RCN toolkit for nurses who are not mental health specialists. Royal College of Nursing. **Publication Code 003 311.**
- Munro (2011).
- Working together to safeguard children (HM Government 2010a).
- Safeguarding children: working together under the Children Act 2004 (2006), Welsh Assembly Government.
- www.nspcc.org.uk (accessed 25 July 2013).
- Independent Safeguarding Authority (ISA) – commenced 1 December 2012.

Strategies for accessing the 'voice of the child'

My premise here is that when health, educational and governmental systems tap into, and are receptive to, this valuable perspective, children's voices will enhance the rights and well-being of children and young people. This is particularly so for children and young people with a developmental condition. The right for the voice of all children to be heard is underpinned by the Human Rights Act (1998) and should be enshrined into the core values of all agencies working with children. Children have a legal right to be heard (e.g. UNCRC (1989/1995); England and Wales, Code of Practice for Special Educational Needs (2002); SENDA (2001); Children Act (1989, 2004)). The Children and Families Bill (2013) demands that assessment and care plans must take into account a child's preferences and views, to capture and explore the meanings that each child assigns to their own experiences. Indeed, the central aims of the CAF involve keeping the child or young person's voice alive and I make the point here that this applies to *all* children, including those who have communication, language and/ or cognitive impairments.

There has been a growing consideration that children are 'are seen as having a perception and experience of childhood that greatly enhances our understanding of childhood in late modernity' (France *et al.* 2000: 151). This 'new approach' to understanding childhood or youth also requires 'methodology that puts the child or young person at the centre of focus' (ibid.). Indeed, a solution that fails to take account of the child's perspective has a reduced chance of meeting the child's needs or of being accepted by the child and therefore being effective.

Three components are seen as crucial to successfully elicit children's responses: a) the situation; b) the sequence of the interview; and c) the questions (Barker 1990).

Interviews should always begin with a general exploration of the child's world and experience. In the first instance, careful face-to-face explanations should introduce the session, followed by enquiry about non-threatening topics. Move onto more sensitive or difficult issues when the child is ready for such questions, and the child will be more likely to cooperate if the opportunity to control the content of the conversation is made clear early on in the interview. Innovation, novelty and ingenuity may be required, but must in no way compromise the validity of the outcome. Working together to safeguard children (HM Government 2006) sets out practice guidance for LSCBs and this document offers a wealth of information to the professional. It also draws attention to the vulnerability of the disabled child as: 'The available UK evidence on the extent of abuse among disabled children suggests that disabled children are at increased risk of abuse and that the presence of multiple disabilities appears to increase the risks of both abuse and neglect' (ibid., Paragraph 11.28).

Eliciting responses in children's interactions is a topic I discuss further in Chapter 7, but I introduce here evidence-based practice demonstrated by Boyden *et al.* (2013). This study found semi-structured questionnaires were effective in the interviewing process, used here to evaluate service provision for young people with a learning disability. However, the use of questionnaires per se carries a note of caution. As Morrow (2001a) argues, questionnaires are useful to identify broad themes or trends, but they cannot elicit the meaning, perspectives and social contexts of behaviours. In addition, the issue of 'acquiescent responding' needs to be considered, where the child or young person gives responses he or she thinks the interviewer wants to hear.

In Chapter 7, I return to this subject in greater depth, and offer strategies that may be useful to access the child's views.

Ethics

A branch of philosophy, ethics, centres on the study of good and bad, right or wrong and endeavours to shape principles or provide a code through which to guide high moral and behavioural standards of professional conduct. Ethical issues abound in the health, education and social care professions and ethical principles are raised elsewhere throughout this book, but in health, education and social care, client vulnerability demands that standards of conduct built on sound ethical foundations are fundamental to practice. Codes of practice aim to safeguard and protect the clients, who must be able to trust those who deal with all matters relating to health and well-being care and, particularly, special education.

Conversely, an ethical code of conduct also protects the professional practitioner and this I discuss later below. Briefly, ethics is about morals and involves giving reasons why it is acceptable to act in a given way in a particular situation. These morals are universal when they concern human welfare and human interests. In the past few decades bioethics, or the study of ways in which science and medicine touch upon our health, our lives, society and our environment, have made an impact, and this can be seen in all human communities, from local to international levels.

It is not my intention here to engage in broad philosophical debate, rather, I briefly introduce two prominent approaches that generally underpinned a framework of standard moral theories in earlier days of medical and health care ethics, and bioethical dilemmas: namely *deontology* and *consequentialist* approaches. At the end of this chapter, I refer to further works from which personal enquiry can be pursued.

The *deontological* approach is based on the premise that an action is right, if your state of mind is right; thus ethics is a matter of choosing which actions are needed, or prohibited, as a matter of duty. The most influential advocate of the approach, Immanuel Kant (1724–1804), saw that there was no basis for self-interest and individual feelings, rather human dignity was the grounding premise. Deontology also refers to a code of ethics for certain professions, such as the medical profession. Human rights are considered a deontological concept and deontological theories are best understood in contrast to *consequentialist* ones.

In contrast then, the *consequentialist* approach is distinguished from deontological ethics because it holds that an action is right, if it can maximize what is desirable in its outcome. The most familiar form is *utilitarianism* where consequences are fundamentally measured in terms of the effects of an action, the ends 'justify the means'; on welfare and happiness of people; or achieving the greatest good for the greatest number of people, a stance advocated by Jeremy Bentham (1748–1832). His use of the term was aligned to the science of morality, and was modified in the principle of utility by John Stuart Mill (1806–1873).

In health services, the Nursing and Midwifery Council (NMC) is the regulator for England, Wales, Scotland and Northern Ireland, upholds standards and ethics, and in practice aims at promoting trust and respect between professionals and their clients (NMC 2011). Failure to observe or comply with this code may bring fitness to practise into question. The NMC regulatory body upholds an ethics code that: acts to safeguard the health and well-being of the public; sets standards and a code of conduct that nurses and midwives are required to follow; ensures that nurses and midwives uphold standards of their professional code; ensures that they are safe to practise; and investigates allegations made against those who may not have abided by the rules of conduct. Basic principles of respect, dignity, confidentiality, care, consent and the need to follow a clear professional code of behaviour are made explicit throughout.

Teaching Standards (DfE 2012b) set a high standard of ethics and behaviour, not only as an expectation, but defined as a part of personal and professional conduct to which professionals must have a regard. Cultural 'ethics' are made clear through the statement of 'Fundamental British Values' (ibid.: 5). These include democracy, the rule of law, individual liberty, mutual respect and tolerance. Establishing a safe environment is also explicitly written into this code. This statutory code clearly sets out professional duties and responsibilities within an ethical framework. Teaching Unions also have a code of professional conduct and ethics that are pretty much in parallel and, in particular, stipulate an ethical code of conduct for teachers and their behaviour and relationships with pupils.

An appropriate working relationship based on mutual respect and trust, well-being and safety, confidentiality and ethical safeguarding processes and practices underpin expectations within all ethical codes. An ethical guide to those concerned with research in education (Hammersley and Traianou 2012) offers five principles that apply equally well to those who teach. They include: minimizing harm; respecting autonomy; protecting privacy; offering reciprocity; and treating people equitably.

The professional body for psychologists in the UK, the British Psychological Society, sets out a code of ethics that their members must abide by, with a Code of Conduct and a series of guidelines for specific activities (Code of Ethics and Conduct 2009). Where a chartered psychologist is found to have behaved in a manner judged as an offence against this code, sanctions according to the seriousness of the transgression serve as a regulatory enforcement of the BPS Code of Ethics.

A code of ethics for social work professionals (BASW 2012) states that ethical awareness is fundamental to the professional practice and integrity of social workers, and that 'ability and commitment to act ethically is an essential aspect of the quality of the service offered to those who engage with social workers' (ibid.: 5). Principles in policy expound on human dignity, respecting rights of self-determination and participation, trustworthiness and maintaining professional boundaries.

Distinct ethical principles common to all codes and guidelines are the need for respect and dignity, a regard for confidentiality, collaboration with those in your care and, most important, informed consent before you begin treatment or care, intervention programmes or when making any decisions that affect the individual.

Many issues have been introduced in this first chapter and the main points I summarize below. The following chapter looks at biological, physical and social models of child development, focusing on developmental progress that is unimpaired and/or monitored within a range of anticipated milestones.

Summary

- Dynamics of the universal, or available to all, health service at any given time is underpinned by fluctuation, adaptation and discontinuation of policies, driven by the political force of the time or government of the day.
- Change is usually in response to prevailing conditions in a community; these can be socially, politically or economically motivated, if not induced by all three variables.
- Legislation serves as the framework for change and service providers at the local level are legally required to develop policy and administration. Systems designated under laws for England have been developed in parallel in other countries that comprise the United Kingdom. Wales, Scotland and Northern Ireland have delegated powers within each of their respective governments or assemblies.
- Key reforms for the past decade have been working towards a model of integrated, multi-agency involvement; emphasis is on supporting the child in the family setting, working with parents/caregivers to deliver integrated services.
- Community-based services, service level agreements and a strengthened health visiting service workforce should work towards health promotion activities, proactive, preventative medical care, rather than reactive practice that responds to need as it arises.
- To better understand the impact of environmental influences within social systems, culture or time frame, they can be examined from a socio-constructivist perspective through a model such as the ecological systems model (Bronfenbrenner 1979).
- A socio-constructivist views disability as a socially defined construct, a social model has now replaced the medical model. Therefore a socially defined construct can, and does, change over time and in social or cultural contexts.
- It is embedded in health, education and social care policy locally, nationally and internationally that the views of the child or young person *must* be accessed by professionals and *always* be taken into account where any decision is being made that affects, or includes, the child.

- Safeguarding and child protection issues are of primary concern to any professional working with children and families, in health, social care or education. Giving due consideration to such issues is an ethical, legal and social demand. Professionals and paraprofessionals in services associated with health and well-being, education, psychology and youth support services have a duty of care to children within their custody.
- Standards embedded in protectionist codes of practice can both ultimately help reduce the risk of abuse or neglect within the family *or* working environment, *and* protect the professional.
- ALL professions produce a code of ethics. Health, education and social care professionals are bound by duty to have a regard of the code that covers their specific professional body. All professionals should be fully cognizant with their profession's code.

Recommended reading and further resources

Useful resource references

Common Assessment Framework for Children and Young People: A Guide for Practitioners (2006). Published by The Children's Workforce Development Council.

Communicating with Children (training courses) NSPCC training course for professionals. Downloaded from https://www.nspcc.org.uk (accessed 29 July 2013).

Department for Education (2006). *Working Together to Safeguard Children*. London, DfE.

Department of Health (DH) (2012). *Getting it Right for Children, Young People and Families*. London, DH.

HM Government (2006). *What to do if You're Worried a Child is Being Abused*. London, HM Government.

UN (2006). *Conventions on the Rights of Persons with Disabilities*. New York, UN.

WHO (2011). World Health Organization (WHO) and the World Bank: World Report on Disability. Geneva, WHO. Downloaded from www.who.int/disabilities/world_report/2011 (accessed 18 July 2013).

Working Together to Safeguard Children. Every Child Matters. Change for Children (2006). Updated 2010, 2013. Downloaded from http://webarchive.nationalarchives.gov.uk/20130401151715/https://www.education.gov.uk/publications/eOrderingDownload/WT2006%20Working_together.pdf (accessed 19 December 2013).

Further recommended resources

Ethics and philosophy

An introductory guide that is user friendly is:

Jill Oliphant (Author) and Jon Mayled (ed.) (2007). *OCR Religious Ethics for AS and A2*. Oxon, Routledge.

Warburton, N. (2004). *Philosophy: The Basics* (4th edn). London, Routledge. In particular Chapter 2: 'Right and wrong', pp. 39–66.

Chapter 2   Child development, reviews and screening

Intended learning outcomes

At the end of this chapter you will

- know the key features presented in prominent models of child development;
- understand the social constructivist influence on child development theory of both Piaget and Vygotsky;
- understand principles of attachment theory, transition stages, adolescence and influences that serve to shape the identity and personality and develop the individual's locus of control (LoC);
- know the features of a psychosocial framework that views development as a lifelong cycle;
- understand the basic structures and functions of the regions of the brain;
- understand how in early child development interactions and environmental experiences impact on biological and physiological features of the brain;
- understand crucial *normal* developmental changes during the formative early years of children's lives, the foundation years, from pregnancy to age five;
- be able to make the distinction between screening and diagnostic assessment procedures; and
- understand, as an allied professional working with children and families, the fundamental principles of ethical codes of behaviour.

Key words (see glossary)

Atypical, cognition.

Key words (defined in the text)

Adolescence, attachment, axon, brain stem, cerebellum, cerebrum, dendrite, deoxyribonucleic acid (DNA), frontal lobe, genetic, identity, locus of control (LoC), longitudinal study, medulla oblongata, naturalistic setting, plasticity, pons, screening, self-efficacy, social constructivist, social learning theory, surveillance, synapse.

Introduction

In order to understand atypical or anomalous development in the child, the first priority for professionals is to understand typical or age-related development patterns. In this chapter, the key concepts in prominent models of typical, or normal, child development are described. I start by introducing the primary stages of development that Piaget posits, generally acknowledged as being, in its time, a radically different approach to the study of child development. I then bring together concepts from the social constructivist perspective to contextualize the influence of both Piaget and Vygotsky on developmental theory.

In this chapter, a socio-cultural view of the development of cognition (Vygotsky 1978) is summarized, and significant features of attachment theory are highlighted (Bowlby 1951; Ainsworth *et al.* 1978). The development of the individual's identity, shaped during the transition through adolescence, is then presented, and prominent social learning theory described (Bandura 1977, 1982, 1989/1992). Consideration is then given to identity development and self-agency and LoC, both believed to be factors that contribute to the shaping of personality (Rotter 1966, 1990). Major biological, educational and social transitions in adolescence are explored, and given context in the eight-stage framework of Erikson's psychosocial model of development or a lifelong cycle (Erikson 1980/1994). Following this, I describe in broad terms early neurophysiological and structural anatomy of the brain, and its development. Subsequent functioning attributed to specific regions of the brain are also identified (Blakemore and Choudhury 2006).

The concepts of surveillance and screening are introduced and the significant time points are highlighted from pre-birth to young adulthood. The chapter closes with the return to the issue of ethics introduced in the last chapter, but contextualized here within the issue of genetic information, screening pre-birth and/or genetic counselling in specific conditions or disorders.

As Chapter 1 has shown, conceptions of childhood, not only in Britain, are changing, and an emerging body of research attends to the meaning that children are participants in the construction of their own development (Smith and Taylor 2000). Viewed from a socio-cultural perspective, and in an earlier time frame, the position of children has looked at the social and cultural context wherein the developing child is placed. Within this field the construction central to theory in developed countries is a model of the child as in need of protection by adults. Further, that adults structure the environment to foster learning they deem most important to children. This view is implicit in the work of Piaget's staged model of cognitive development.

One of the foremost psychologists, generally considered a leading force in the study of child development, Piaget's (1896–1980) powerful theory of stages in cognitive development revolutionized the way the process of development was framed. The four-stage model he proposed was linked loosely to physiological developmental stages, and acknowledged by psychologists and educationalists as a model through which to understand cognition and development. Such views, from the stance of a positivist or scientific observer, have carried an enduring influence on societal conceptions of childhood. This model also reinforces perceptions of children as being dependent, irrational and vulnerable for a substantial period of time. This belief has since been challenged (Donaldson 1987) and much of Piaget's work has since been overtaken in many areas by further developmental theories.

Key concepts of Piaget's theory

Piaget conducted naturalistic research, observing behaviour in a natural setting, to understand child development, and coined the term 'genetic epistemology'. This describes how he considered knowledge developed in the child and he proposed that children's thinking, or cognition, does not develop smoothly. Rather, there are transition points whereby the child moves into a new area of development and is thus able to master new capabilities. Implicit was that understanding develops in a linear fashion.

Piaget's theories view that three factors underlie development: genes, developmental history and current environment, and, over time, much debate has arisen about the role of these factors, alone, and in combination with each other. His theories are individualistic in emphasis, and stress that the child's adaptation to the physical world and growth results in logical and mathematical thinking. Piaget's theories did advance constructivist theory about knowledge, advocating that it is constructed through active engagement between individuals and the world wherein they are placed, but little consideration was given to the processes of social transmission of knowledge from one generation to the next. I summarize here Piaget's central assumptions and key ideas.

Assumptions

- To understand behaviour, it is necessary to consider inner mental concepts such as thoughts, beliefs and cognitive structures.
- Mental concepts change over time through childhood and these changes hold a major influence on people's behaviour, judgement and attitudes at different ages.
- The environment should provide a context for children to explore, which in turn leads to cognitive growth.

Key premises

- Development is homogenous regardless of the child's culture.
- Intellectual development occurs as a process in stages.
- Constructivist underpinning: individuals construct their own knowledge and understanding of their world in response to their experiences.

Key concepts defined

- Object permanence – a young infant is unable to realize objects in the world exist permanently, even when he or she is not around.
- Centration and egocentrism are the beliefs that you are the centre of the universe, and all will revolve around you.
- Representation – internal knowledge is conceptualized as a model of external reality.

Universal stages

- The Sensorimotor Period – from 0–2 years approximately.
- Pre-operational – approximately age 2–7 years.
- Concrete operations – approximately age 7–11 years.
- Formal operations – approximately age 12 years onwards (see Table 2.1).

TABLE 2.1 Piaget's stages of cognitive development

Stage		Characterized by
Stage 1	Sensorimotor (0–2 years)	Egocentrism – the child cannot distinguish between itself and its environment Object permanence – aware that things continue to exist even when no longer present
Stage 2	Pre-operational (2–7 years)	Class inclusion problems, understands simple classification but subsets of categorization not mastered Egocentrism – child still not understanding that all others do not see, think or feel things the same as him/her Lack of conservation – the inability to realize that some things remain constant or unchanged even though they may change in appearance. Child fails to conserve properties such as number or substance Centration – a tendency to focus on only one aspect of a problem or object
Stage 3	Concrete operational (7–11 years)	Operations – can carry out mental operations logically, manipulate information Achieves conservation of number and weight Classifies objects according to several features or order in a series
Stage 4	Formal operational (12 onwards)	Logically thinks abstract thoughts Reasoning/deduction – mental structures allow internalized manipulation of problems Decentration – systematic deductive reasoning, attending to more than one thing at a time

What does the child build?

- **Schemata** – basic building blocks of intelligent behaviour. Internal representations of specific physical or mental action that continue to develop and increase in complexity.
- **Operations** – acquired developmentally, higher order mental structures that lead the child to understand more complex rules about how the environment works. Logical manipulations that deal with the relationship between schemata.

How does the child build?

- **Adaptation** – adapting to the world through assimilation and accommodation.
- **Assimilation** – the process where new objects, situations or ideas are understood through the schemata the child already possesses. The world fits around what the child already knows.
- **Intrinsic motivation** – children are intrinsically motivated, not motivated by extrinsic rewards from adults.
- **Accommodation** – the process where existing schemata have to be modified to fit new situations, objects or information. Schemata are expanded or new ones are created.

Methods of investigation

- **Observation** – Piaget's naturalistic setting of child's interactions and play.
- **Diaries (longitudinal study)** – Piaget studied his own children over time, recorded changes in a diary of noted events.
- **Experimentation** – e.g. cross-sectional experiments comparing the ability of two different age groups on the conservation task.

Limitations, advances and challenges

- Theory of cognitive development based on high socio-economic population/own children, difficult to generalize findings to a larger population.
- He made observations but failed to explain causal processes.
- Failed to take account of the developing child's environmental factors.
- Challenged over linear movement through stages: model at best is a useful approximation.
- Major changes in development (3–4 months and again 7–8 months) aligned to changes in brain structure and functions since identified.
- Insufficient consideration of language acquisition and development.

Key concepts in Vygotsky's development theory

Social learning theories, and in particular those of Vygotsky, make clear the influence of the parent or caregiver in the shaping of learning mastery and of self-perceptions (Vygotsky 1978). The key notion of this developmental theory is that as adults we have the ability to think, and reason is itself the outcome of a fundamentally social process. Infants, and later children, are primarily social beings that are able to engage with others, but able to do very little for themselves.

As with Piaget, Vygotsky viewed the process of development as a series of stages the child moves through, but it diverges from there. Vygotsky's model posits that at the initial stage the child is unable to do certain things unaided, but as they move through the process, the child is able to do things *with others*, so that by the final stage, the child is able to do things for him or herself. Thus the developing child's level of ability was seen not in terms of what s/he *could* do, rather what s/he was capable of when help was given. This describes the concept of a *zone of proximal* (or the next) development. It takes account of the role of teaching, and the teaching–learning process, as a social exchange wherein shared meanings are built up through joint activity.

Family influence, attitudes and relationships begin the formation process in early years, and the reactions of significant others in the child's life are thus considered an important influence on how self-perceptions and self-esteem evolve. Moving on then into adolescence, peer relations become more intense and extensive. Peer comparison increases (Coleman and Hendry 1990) and with peer approval often being sought over parents' approval. Several developmental changes at this time will also serve to alter attitudes, motivation and the manner in which adolescents interact with both peers and family.

Vygotsky's key concepts

- Children construct knowledge.
- Education and social interaction influence cognitive development.
- Learning can lead the development process.
- Development cannot be separated from the social context of development.
- Language plays a central role in cognitive development.
- The level of assisted performance is the maximum the child can achieve with help.
- Zone of Proximal Development (ZPD) describes the difference between the level of independent performance and the level of assisted performance.
- Our social and cultural development context determines the content and processes of our thought.

Vygotsky proposed that language and thought began as separate processes but gradually converged and influenced each other. He saw speech as a social tool with which to interact with others; at around the age of two years, language and thought begin to converge. Then language becomes more meaningful and more easily understood. Thus language is used to communicate thoughts to others publicly, and privately directs or monitors thoughts. Initially at this stage though, the child may do this aloud, or through 'egocentric speech'. Through maturation, egocentric speech still directs learning but becomes 'internalized'.

Limitations and challenges

- Insufficient research from Vygotsky to support his ideas.
- Inaccessibility of consciousness to observation makes investigation 'non-scientific'.
- Vygotsky's death at a young age and the reliance on translations of his work has inherent limitations. However, both constructivism and social constructivism studies, based on his work, have taken his theories to a new and different level.

Attachment theory

Attachment theory has a focus of interest in developmental psychology and refers to the emotional bonding attachment and enduring close emotional bonds with another person. In the neonate, the first attachments are between the infant and the mother. Attachment theories developed through a plethora of research in the 1960s and 1970s but what was developed then still holds some value in modernity, and even with different child-rearing patterns that are present in developed societies today.

Originated by Bowlby (1951) in line with Darwin's theory of natural selection, the underlying premise thus sees any behaviour that helps the infant survive, reach maturity and reproduce itself will, it is presumed, be maintained in the gene pool. A theoretical descriptive and explanatory framework, derived through ethological, or scientific, study, offers greater understanding of the primary interrelationship between caregiver and baby. There is some crossover between more notable theories and theoretical concepts in later developed models of identified attachment processes, the theories and concepts of which are broadly summarized in Table 2.2.

TABLE 2.2 Theories and concepts of attachment in infancy

Theorist	Concepts and characteristics
Bowlby (1951) (naturalistic observations)	Maternal deprivation hypothesis Monotrophy – close bond with one figure 'Critical period' for mothering
Bowlby et al. (1956)	Internal working model Proximity maintenance Safe haven Secure base Separation distress Attachment behaviour instinctive – motivational system – attachment behavioural system Affectionless psychopathy
Schaffer and Emerson (1964)	Three distinct stages of attachment Indiscriminate attachment (0–6 weeks) Specific attachment (six weeks to seven months) Multiple attachments
Ainsworth and Bell (1969)	'Strange situation' technique Type A: avoidant-anxious
Ainsworth et al. (1978)	Type B: secure Type C: resistant-ambivalent
Main and Solomon (1990)	Type D: disorganized/inconsistent; added to the pattern of attachments shown in maltreated children
Rutter (1972)	Privation Disruption Distortion

Bowlby (ibid.) revolutionized thinking about a child's tie to the mother and its disruption through separation, deprivation or bereavement, or being denied emotional comfort. He characterized attachment as interaction patterns that develop in order to fulfil the needs and emotional development of the infant. This bias of attachment to one figure is a characteristic he termed *monotropism* and conceptualized it as being a vital bond with one figure, usually the mother or primary caregiver, a concept that has since been argued against (Bowlby 1969; Ainsworth et al. 1978; Donaldson 1987; Main and Solomon 1990). As the theory developed, it was suggested that the infant is born with an innate primary instinctive need to form an emotional bond with the mother or caregiver. This attachment differs in kind from attachments to other subsidiary figures and, importantly, it also serves as an internal working model for other relationships throughout later life.

This model he viewed as comprising cognitive representations, or schema, based on the day-to-day interactions with the primary caregiver that persist relatively unchanged throughout life, and act as a guide or prototype for all future social relationships (Bowlby 1969). His exposition laid great emphasis on attachment security, and an expectation that key persons will be available and supportive in times of need.

Important was the suggestion that a primary caregiver must be a constant for a crucial period in the first years of the infant's life, and that this should occur within a critical period of time (approximately by the age of 30 months). Underpinning the maternal deprivation hypothesis that Bowlby postulated was that crucially a failure to initiate, or a maternal attachment breakdown, would be detrimental to the child's mental health in later life. However, there is a lack of supporting evidence for this claim and the view has since been modified (Rutter 1972) to show that the breadth of attachments is largely determined by social settings. While Bowlby's ideas of attachment were important, research has shown since that multiple attachments can be formed and within a sensitive time period (ibid.).

Attachment behaviours function like a fixed pattern and all share the same purpose in a dyadic or two-person relationship. The infant initiates contact through signals, or innate social releaser behaviour, such as crying and smiling, to which the caregiver instinctively responds. Thus the child's behaviour creates a reciprocal pattern of interaction. The concept of reciprocity is raised throughout this book, and in different contexts, but reciprocity in this context refers to the interactions between the mother or caregiver and the infant. This is explored further in a case study of the Solihull Approach (SA) presented later in this book (see Chapter 8). Adaptive behaviour described in attachment theory is seen as an aid to survival particularly as attachment provides food, security and a safe base from which to explore and understand the world. The effects of attachment can be seen when the infant and the attachment figure are separated and this, Bowlby (1951) postulated, operated across different cultures and was thus universal in babies. He saw distress at separation as following a pattern of *infant protest*, following with *despair* and ending in *eventual detachment*. The concept of separation anxiety, derived in part from animal studies, influenced his view that the significant period of attachment between 1–5 years needs to be stable if emotional and intellectual problems in adulthood were to be avoided.

Attachment has been investigated using the *strange situation* technique (Schaffer and Emerson 1964) that measured the strength of attachments by *separation anxiety*, or how *distressed* the child became when separated from the main caregiver, and *stranger anxiety* that showed the distress shown by the infant when left alone with an unfamiliar person. Their conclusion was that human attachments develop in three distinct phases given in Table 2.2. These describe the strength of attachments developmentally; suggest attachment is formed between 6–8 months; and suggest the higher the mother's emotional responsiveness the stronger the attachment. Significantly by 18 months of age, very few infants studied were attached to only one person, and some infants had formed five or more attachments.

A technique devised to investigate patterns of attachment by a colleague of Bowlby's, Mary Ainsworth, was the *strange situation* experiment (Ainsworth *et al.* 1978). Using this laboratory paradigm, all infants were presented with a standardized, controlled and replicable set of experiences. The different outcomes were attributed to the infant possessing different predispositions for behaviours related to attachment, and the predispositions believed to have been primarily gained from the infant's particular experiences with their carer over the previous year. Based on observation, three major styles of attachment were identified:

- secure attachment;
- ambivalent-insecure attachment; and
- avoidant-insecure attachment.

A fourth attachment style known as *disorganized-insecure* attachment was later added (Main and Solomon 1990). Numerous studies over the years have supported these conclusions, and later additional research has shown that these early attachment styles can help predict behaviours later in life. Attachment theorists have found that people characteristically exhibit one of three attachment styles: secure, anxious secure or avoidant. Those individuals with secure attachment styles are more likely to focus on the other, experience compassion and are helpful to others, regardless of whether the recipient is their own child or not (Crowell and Feldman 1988; Crowell and Feldman 1991); a romantic partner (Carnelley *et al.* 1996); or a stranger (Mikulincer *et al.* 2003).

Concepts and assertions in Bowlby's theory of attachment

- *Monotropy*: the vital and close bond to one attachment figure.
- A child has an innate or inborn need to attach to one main attachment figure.
- Concept of *monotropy* underpinned maternal deprivation hypothesis.
- Advocated the child should receive continuous care, from one carer, and this is the most important figure in the first two years of life.
- If attachment figure is broken or disrupted during that two-year period, the infant is at risk of eventual mental health problems.
- Long-term consequences of maternal deprivation may lead to delinquency, depression or affectionless psychopathy.

Summary of attachment characteristics

- **Safe haven** – reliable caregiver gives comfort at times whenever feeling threatened or afraid.
- **Secure base** – caregiver provided reliable foundation to support child as s/he develops.
- **Proximity maintenance** – child explores the world but stays close to caregiver, e.g. strong caregiver–child relationship during adolescence.
- **Separation distress** – child upset or unhappy when separated from caregiver.

Attachment styles extended from Bowlby's theory

- **Secure attachment** – securely attached to caregivers, happy when caregivers are around, secure feelings that caregiver will return.
- **Ambivalent attachment** – infant ambivalently attached; feels caregiving may be unreliable, not wholly trusting of caregiver.
- **Avoidant attachment** – infant tends to keep away from parent, distrust caregiver, observable style may be seen in neglected or abused infants.
- **Disorganized attachment** – no clear or mixed attachment, caregiver may be apprehensive *and* reassuring but inconsistently and infant is confused and untrusting.

In summary, the concept of attachment is considered to be what:

- lays the foundation for emotional and cognitive growth;
- is there to ensure the survival of the child;
- defines the affectionate bond between two individuals that endures time and distance;

- joins two people emotionally;
- is fundamental to emotional, social, physical and cognitive development;
- promotes resilience to trauma, disadvantage or deprivation in later life;
- fosters attunement in the interaction between the child and the parent/carer;
- can influence a child's attainment to his/her full cognitive potential;
- influences the development of a healthy sense of self;
- underpins the development of emotional intelligence (Goleman 1996) and empathy (discussed again in Chapter 9).

Activity 2.1: SAQs

- What is meant by the term 'attachment'?
- Observation in a *strange situation* has been used to investigate cultural variations in attachment. Give one advantage of using observation in psychological research.
- How does behaviour of securely attached infants differ from that of insecurely attached infants?
- What do you understand by the concept of 'reciprocity'?
- What is 'naturalistic observation'? Name one advantage and one disadvantage.

Adolescence and social learning theory

Adolescence is usually thought of as a period of transition, a time of both change and consolidation, with major physical changes that impact the sense of self and intellectual growth. Additionally, the changes in role demanded of young people at this time also make demands in terms of modifications of the self-concept. Developmentally this stage is a crucial and formative stage for the development of self-worth, where success is paramount to success academically, socially and physically, and a period where failure can result in isolation and loneliness. During this social transition, adolescents spend more time with peers rather than parents, however the role of parents or carers as well as the family during this period is also crucial.

Studies have shown that when compared to individuals from step-families or blended families, individuals from the traditional, intact biological families tend to fare better emotionally, socially, physically and psychologically (Carpenter 2000; Love and Murdock 2004). Elsewhere adolescent perceptions of secure attachment to both birth parents and peers have been found to be associated with high scores on a measure of self-perceived strengths (Raja *et al*. 1992). 'Traditional' family values are described here as comprising blood relatives and safety nets for the aged, infirm or other kin with a need, although as noted elsewhere (Mitterauer and Seider 1983) in the developed world, such a stereotyped notion of 'the family' with traditional values, two married parents of the opposite gender and with planned children, is arguably the reality for very few families in the twenty-first century.

Moving out from the family interaction setting, in adolescent psychology, belonging and acceptance in the form of social group membership at this time is considered an important influence on the developing self (Ausubel 2002) and underpins self/social development theory (Bandura 1989/1992). The goal of such social interactions is given as a need to identify with peer groups and foster peer acceptance, however for the adolescent affected by mood swings, unable to comprehend social cues or presenting with social clumsiness attributable to a specific disorder, the normal social uncertainties associated with this developmental age are even greater.

For the young person with a developmental impairment or debilitating condition, the opportunity for membership, or inclusion, in social groups may be denied them, particularly where independent functioning is an issue. In this developmental period, normally developing adolescents are sensitive to peer rejection, or exclusion from a particular clique or group. For the young person with a disorder or disability, this may exacerbate feelings of social isolation and at worst impact on their mental health. It is therefore essential that parents, carers and professionals take account of how the developmental effect will undoubtedly compound psychosocial and emotional functioning during this period. The discussion of these issues I expand upon later (see Chapter 6).

Social learning theory (Bandura 1989/1992), or social cognitive theory, focuses on the shaping of personality by social experience and observational learning. It emphasizes the lifelong development process and takes account of different types and patterns of change. Of interest here is the role of the social dimension in child development and the central tenet of the model that holds that children develop through learning from other events and people around them, or through an observational learning model. Thus all behaviour is learned through the child's interactions and experiences in the developmental environment. The model also accounts for how the young child may acquire many novel responses in a large number of settings, and with both negative and positive consequences.

Bandura (ibid.: 4) set out the notion of 'reciprocal causation' that sees continuum learning as the whole range of behaviours, desirable and undesirable, through the processes of observation and imitation. Different sources of influence, or reciprocal causation, are presumed to have different impacts that occur at different times. They are presumed to impact at different strengths and activate reciprocal influence over time, and once again the concept of reciprocal transactions is drawn into a model of development. Here influences in Bandura's (ibid.) model are considered to be bidirectional, and reciprocal, and are both concepts that underpin Bronfenbrenner's (1979) ecological systems introduced in the previous chapter.

Implicit in the model is that individuals develop and modify expectations, beliefs, emotions and learned competencies through social influences, modelling, instruction and social persuasion (Bandura 1986). Significant here however is that much social learning is incidental and acquired through observing actual behaviour, and seeing the consequences of that behaviour for others. Social learning theory has often been used to explain the intergenerational transmission of aggression, or the cycle of violence, although also criticized as offering an oversimplified description of human behaviour in that it fails to take sufficient account of either inheritance factors or the role of maturation in development.

While aligned to many of the concepts of traditional learning theory, Bandura added a further element. This viewed external environmental reinforcement as only one factor in the child's development and suggested that an intrinsic self-reflective capability also operates. It is hypothesized that this mechanism gives the individual the capacity to both analyse their experience and to think about one's own thought processes, through a 'self-efficacy' mechanism that Bandura (1994) suggests plays a central role in human agency. Basically then, it involves self-judgement of one's personal capabilities, or a constant appraisal of one's self-efficacy.

As such, the response of others towards the individual's actions or behaviour would be a crucial dimension of the self-efficacy process and the family, significant others and peer relationships can be presumed to play an important role in self-efficacy development.

Epstein (1990) too stresses the importance of familial sources of self-efficacy asserting that parents contribute to their children's intellectual growth by: preparing the child for school; placing a value on education; and conveying belief in their child's scholastic ability. Initial efficacy experience can therefore be considered as centred in the family, but expanding as the child's social world expands. Perceived self-efficacy can also serve to promote health and well-being living, and a strong perception of self-regulatory efficacy to effect change will positively affect personal change whatever the phase in life. The weaker the perceptions of self-efficacy, the less likely it is that a child will have a robust, self-confident positive personality, but rather they may be more vulnerable and prone to anxiety, stress and the negative consequences that such a state manifests on normal developmental processes.

Sources of self-efficacy

- Mastery experiences success.
- Through the vicarious experiences that are provided by social models.
- Social persuasion.
- Modification of self-beliefs of efficacy that can reduce people's stress reactions and change negative emotions.

Effects of low self-efficacy

- Depression and anxiety – through unfulfilled aspiration.
- Impact on self-efficacy of biological systems that affect healthy functions.
- Stress – weak sense of efficacy, failure to exercise control over stressors, activates autonomic reactions. Impairing immune functions.

Efficacy-activated processes

- Cognitive processes: thinking processes involved in the acquisition, organization and use of information.
- Motivation: activation to action.
- Affective processes: processes regulating emotional states and elicitation of emotional reactions.
- Perceived self-efficacy: individual's belief about their capabilities to produce effects.
- Self-regulation: exercise of influence over one's own motivation, thought processes, emotional states and patterns of behaviour.

(Bandura 1994: 71–74)

Social learning theory: 'locus of control'

In social learning theory, 'personality' represents an interaction of the individual with his or her environment, and within psychology locus of control (LoC) is considered an important aspect of personality that bridges theories found in both behavioural and cognitive psychology. The central tenet of Rotter's (1954) LoC theory holds that an individual's perception about the underlying main causes of events will determine the outcome of events in his or her life. It views behaviour as being guided by reinforcements of reward or punishment; indeed the construct was initially coined as 'Locus of Control of Reinforcement'. It was through such contingencies that Rotter thought individuals come to hold beliefs about what causes their actions (Rotter 1954, 1966).

Conceptualized as a continuum ranging from *internal* to *external*, the theory holds that individuals described as *internal* will continue to strive for the effects or outcome that they want, using their best efforts, or drawing on intrinsic motivation, to attain their goal. Alternatively an *external* would regard the outcome to be influenced by chance, luck or outside factors, or extrinsic motivation, and beyond their control or influence (Lefcourt 1982). The point has been made (Maines and Robinson 2001: 6) that 'we may hypothesize that externals are less likely to strive for achievements which they do not believe to be dependent on his or her own efforts'. Put in the context of self-esteem, a positive correlation has been found between *internality*, robust self-esteem and achievement (Lawrence 1996).

Placing LoC theory in context alongside the tenets of Bandura's (1994) theories that argue individuals' beliefs in their efficacy can regulate their learning, will influence the mastery of academic activities and can determine aspirations, levels of motivation and academic accomplishments. The need becomes apparent to identify some of the many sources of influence that impact on the holistic shaping of the child throughout its development. Here I again draw attention to the value of using the aforementioned ecological system model developed by Bronfenbrenner.

A psychosocial 'lifelong cycle' model

Historically, an implicit view was that the process of development, from birth, through pre-school to school age was complete by adolescence; a view that has been modified over time, with research taking account of the physical growth and change from puberty onwards (Coleman and Hendry 1990).

The notion that the brain continues to develop during adolescence has now entered the public domain, as have descriptions about how these ongoing changes may at least partially underlie stereotypical adolescent behaviours such as risk taking in the presence of peers, mood swings, volatile outbursts, sleeping late and thrill seeking (Morgan 2005). Advancements in neuroscience support physiological changes that parallel periods of observed behavioural change, showing us that neural pathways and synapses continue to change over life's course, with more intense periods of change occurring with developmental periods of change such as adolescence. This process, termed neuroplasticity, also confirms that the brain, as a physiological organ, is not static and that throughout life the brain can, and does, change.

A model taking account of lifelong maturation is offered by Erikson (1980/1994) and based on the premise that we continue to alter our image of ourselves, and we learn how to react, and interact, with others as we grow older and experience a wider range of relationships. Erikson's model suggests that stages of development are aligned to psychoanalytic theories such as those given in Freud's ideas. He challenged the view that the first five years of life are not the only years that have implications for later development, but that developmental stages continue throughout life's span. Erikson's (ibid.) model is a developmental plan wherein personality develops according to a determined series of steps. It focuses on strengths that develop within each stage, and the model fits from the cradle to grave or from birth through to maturity and death. It is also noted here that this model is a framework for healthy, 'normal' or unimpaired development.

The model posits that changes occur as a response to the impact of social experience across a whole lifespan and through eight stages that are summarized in Table 2.3. It is characterized as the individual passing through each stage, although mastery in one stage is not a requirement before moving on to the next stage. It takes account of the interaction with biological and socio-cultural influences, and the encountering of conflicting influences. Erikson (ibid.) proposed that at each stage associated positive and negative counterbalancing tasks or crises are encountered (e.g. Stage 1 – *trust* versus *mistrust*). If the individual is to achieve full potential in the next stage, each has to be achieved.

To elaborate, stage one of Erikson's model would see the infant as being totally dependent on the caregiver and the development of 'trust' would be based on the dependability and the quality of that primary caregiver. If the child develops trust he will feel safe and secure in the world. However, where the caregiver is inconsistent, or emotionally unavailable or rejecting, this would contribute to feelings of mistrust in the infant. As a result, the child will fail to develop trust but, instead, will develop feelings of fear, mistrust and a belief that the world is an inconstant and unpredictable environment. I return to this model in Chapter 5 when discussing disorders on the autism spectrum and again when discussing the psychosocial and emotional impact of a developmental disorder in Chapter 6.

Key concepts

- Basic conflicts are counterbalanced through positive and negative crises.
- Caregiver's anxiety will be transferred to the infant.
- Inconsistent care does not allow the infant to develop a sense of trust.
- A child needs to feel safe and protected from harm in order to explore its environment.
- Neglect or abuse lessens attempts to communicate and delays motor development.
- Three components contribute to sense of ego identity: biology, individual psychology and social surroundings.
- Ego identity as awareness of sameness, and difference, in relations with others.
- Ego synthesis is viewed as child's way of mastering their own experience.

Basic opposing conflicts in each of the eight stages

1. Trust – mistrust.
2. Autonomy – shame and doubt.
3. Initiative – guilt.
4. Industry – inferiority.

5   Identity – role confusion.
6   Intimacy – isolation.
7   Generativity – stagnation.
8   Ego integrity – despair.

(Erikson 1980/1994)

TABLE 2.3 Eight stages of development adapted from those described by Erikson (1980)

Psychosocial stage	Crises of each stage	Significant events	Consequence
Infancy 0–18 months	Trust vs mistrust	Feeding	Success: a sense of trust if caregivers give reliable care, loving and consistent care. Failure: a lack of reliable care will lead to mistrust.
Early years 2–3 years	Autonomy vs shame and doubt	Toilet training	Success: develops a sense of personal control over physical skills and a sense of independence and positive autonomy. Failure: feelings of shame and self-doubt.
Pre-school 3–5 years	Initiative vs guilt	Exploration	Beginning to assert control over their environment. Success: a strong sense of purpose. Too many expressions of power will lead to adult disapproval. Result: feelings of guilt.
School age 6–11 years	Industry vs inferiority	School and academic	A need to cope with changing social and learning situations. Success: feelings of competence. Failure: connected to feelings of inferiority.
Adolescence 12–18 years	Identity vs role confusion	Social relationships	Develops sense of self, ego identity and social identity. Success: well-adjusted young person. Failure: weak sense of self, role confusion.
Young adulthood 19–40 years	Intimacy vs isolation	Relationships and life partnerships	Forms intimate, loving relationships. Success: strong relationships. Failure: loneliness and isolation.
Middle adulthood 40–65 years	Generativity vs stagnation	Work and parenthood	Create or nurture outlasting change or social benefit. Success: children; creating change to improve life for others. Failure: shallow involvement in community or society.
Maturity 60 years to death	Ego integrity vs despair	Reflection on life	Looking for a sense of fulfilment. Success: feelings of wisdom. Peaceful reflection. Failure: regret, bitterness and despair.

Social identity theories and self-categorization

Identity formation processes that begin to synthesize during puberty and adolescent years are carried on throughout the years of adult life. Through studies on the role of the self-categorization process, it has been suggested that as with concepts such as self-esteem and self-efficacy, people attain part of their self-esteem from their group memberships and that peer influence reinforces group behaviours to effect conformity to the behaviours stereotypically associated with a particular group (Tajfel and Turner 1986).

The role of the pre-school, early years and formal education as an agent for developing a shared social identity and self-efficacy is one that cannot be ignored. In the early years context, these settings function as a primary place for the development of social and cognitive validation of self-efficacy. It has also been suggested that group behaviour is simply individuals acting in terms of a shared social identity. The benefit or underlying motivations for social categorization theory can thus be presumed to be the enhancement of self-esteem through shared group behaviours (Turner and Oakes 1989).

Activity 2.2: SAQs

- How do the physical changes in puberty contribute to identity shaping in early adolescence?
- What cultural influences help, or hinder, the shaping of identity for the child with a developmental disorder or learning difficulties?
- What information about development will the ecological systems approach add to your understanding of adolescence, from the perspective of developmental psychology?
- Name three influences that shape self-identity.
- What is meant by the terms 'ego-identity' and 'ego-synthesis'?

The developing brain: significant structures

To understand the complexities of how nature and nurture interact, developmental theories need to sit alongside physiological and neurological development. In normal development the brain, as it matures, adapts the body to the environment through the process of reinforcing connections between nerve cells that are most advantageous to the individual. In the twenty-first century, we know much more about not only how the brain functions, but how experiences are laid down. It is acknowledged that there are critical periods for brain development, and early experiences can have a direct impact on the brain wiring process and longer-term behaviours, even before maturation has taken place.

It has been advocated that training for HVs should include a strong focus on the early brain development at the pre-natal, infant and early years of the child, particularly if they are to understand infant and adolescent mental health (Wilson *et al.* 2008). Knowing how the brain develops is also essential for understanding how the brain functions in normal development, and which areas of functions are impaired in congenital developmental disorders. Through the discipline of cognitive neuroscience we are beginning to understand better how the young brain develops, and how the mature brain continues to learn. Research has also shown us that the human brain is susceptible to sensitive periods, notably in the first year of life, but still so in puberty and adolescence (Blakemore and Choudhury 2006).

From the embryo to the adult stage, the brain evolves and with advances in technology and particularly cognitive neuroscience (see Chapter 3), it is possible to map the structure, observe first hand the brain performing functions and understand processes involved in cognitive functioning, or how individuals learn. We also now know that the human brain has plasticity, a property that allows it to alter its biological, chemical and physical properties. As the brain changes, functions and behaviour are modified in parallel and the cerebral alterations at the genetic or synaptic level are brought about by a variety of factors encountered in the developmental environment and through life's experiences.

The hierarchy of the brain structures consist of the **cerebral cortex**, the outermost and top layer of the brain, the most recently evolved and complex part. As you move lower into the brain anatomy, here primitive and basic functions that require less conscious control are situated. The **brain stem**, hindbrain or primitive brain and **limbic system** lie situated above the neck where it connects to the spinal cord, and controls reflexes such as coughing, sneezing or swallowing. Here lie the controls that are responsible for automatic and essential body survival functions such as breathing, blood circulation and the heartbeat. The **mid-brain cerebellum** and limbic system are involved in: emotion, emotional regulation and memory; control over muscle movement, balance and coordination; and control over emotion and impulse, fight or flight responses, blood pressure regulation, hunger, thirst, arousal and sleep.

The **cerebral cortex**, or front brain, is the largest part of the brain, divided into the left and right hemispheres, and connected by the **corpus callosum**, a bundle of nerves and fibres through which information is constantly conveyed across the two hemispheres.

Currents, oscillations and chemicals control brain functions and brain activity, and any imbalance results in dysfunction and/or disorder. Much of what we know about these functions has been inferred from studies of brain damage, trauma and injury, and subtly vindicated through neuroscience imaging techniques (Springer and Deutsch 1997). Lateralization theory of the brain implicates specific functions to the left or right hemisphere with right brain dominance evidenced as traits or strengths in intuitiveness and artistic or creative skills. Left brain dominance, in contrast, is evidenced by strengths in analytical thinking, logic, language and critical thinking.

Brain cells, or neurons, are the foundation of the human brain and these cells communicate with one another via junctions, or synapses, where impulses travel from cell to cell, and support learning and skill development. Motor and sensory neurons relay signals from the brain to the body and messages are coordinated by the **brain stem**, the region of the brain that develops earliest, and connects the **cerebrum** with the spinal cord and comprises also of the **midbrain, medulla oblongata** and the **pons**.

In the child's early years, the brain produces more synapses than it needs and, in response to the child's experience, synaptic activity is fast and disorganized. The brain develops rapidly during early childhood years while attachment behaviours are impacting, and there are critical periods where neglect, stress and trauma can have a profound effect on neurological development. At around the age of two years, some synapses will become strengthened, while ones that are not often used are weakened and trimmed in a pruning process. Pruning is a selective process that is responsive to stimulation through early years sensory experience and peaks by the time the child is aged around three years. Synapses that remain become pathways that are stronger and more efficient and demonstrated in skill competency and established behaviour. This offers one explanation for the phase often termed 'the terrible twos' when the developing child demonstrates self-will, tantrums, temper and outbursts of oppositional behaviour, but when the hard wiring of the most used synaptic connection is made. The **limbic system** is especially significant in processing memory, emotional reactions and impulse, so is an alarm system. Structurally it is located on both sides of the **thalamus**, and under the **cerebrum**, and includes the **hypothalamus** and **amygdala**. The limbic system is interconnected to arousal and pleasure, and influences the endocrine system and the autonomic nervous system. It is thought that the functional maturation of limbic circuits is influenced significantly by early socio-emotional experience.

The last part of the brain to develop is the **cortex** where logic, planning, information processing, perception and cognition occur, and is implicated in reward and decision-making mechanisms. Connected to the limbic system by the **orbitofrontal cortex** that spans, or divides, into two hemispheres, it is here that internal states in the body and external sensory information from the environment are received. The left and right **cerebral hemispheres**, as briefly outlined above, develop in the embryo where the structure and the localization of their functions begin to take shape at approximately only five weeks after conception.

The pathology of the brain is also the powerhouse in memory processing. This is elaborated on further in the following chapter but I summarize here some of the areas of the brain implicated in memory processing. The **cerebellum** not only plays an important role in balance and motor control, but is also involved in the processing of some memories. The **cerebral cortex** of the brain, divided into four major lobes, plays the key role in memory, perceptual awareness and attention. The **pre-frontal cortex** plays an important role in processing short-term memories and retaining information or storing longer-term memories. The **parietal lobe** is involved in integrating sensory information from various senses, the **temporal lobe** utilizes sensory information, processes visual and semantic information, and is a key player in long-term memory, and the **medial temporal lobe** is thought to be involved in the declarative and episodic memory.

The brain develops from pre-birth to adolescence and from the time of conception a combination of genes and external factors interplay in the infant. This affects how genes are expressed, and how brain connections are formed. While we now know the brain has plasticity and remains capable of change throughout life, the critical period when the most significant changes are occurring is the first few years of life. This is when the brain is at its most vulnerable. The foundation of neural structures in the frontal lobes is not fully developed until early adulthood, although the basic architecture is constructed throughout this developmental period through early experiences, both negative and positive. It is thus a critical time in the development of children's brains and their psychosocial functioning in later life.

Myelination in brain development refers to the process whereby brain cells and brain systems grow and develop through use-dependent neurological processes that are built on through use. Several use-dependent chemical and structural growth processes take place in a typical brain cell or neuron. Comprising of several parts, of which the cell body, axon and dendrites work collectively, they trigger synaptic activity or 'jump' between the small gaps between cells in a network. A fatty covering that grows along the axon, called myelin, acts as an insulator, and massively increases the speed of the action along the length of the axon. Thus the exchange of information within the neurological network is faster and more efficient. When a brain cell is activated it increases the rate that myelination takes place, and thus the phrase 'use it or lose it' can be best understood.

Structural maturation of neurons and the connecting pathways is required for successful cognitive, motor and sensory functions in the developing child. Importantly, sensory and motor brain regions become fully myelinated in the first few years of life. Although the volume of brain tissue remains stable, axons in the frontal cortex continue to be myelinated well into adolescence (Blakemore and Choudhury 2006). At around the same time as the language areas become active, myelination occurs on the pre-frontal lobes. Here the child begins to develop self-consciousness, suggesting the emergence of an internal executor that plays a major role in maintaining attention. Usually frontal lobes do not become fully myelinated until full adulthood because certain brain areas take many years to mature. This however offers one explanation as to why young people and young adults are more emotional and impulsive than older, more mature adults.

At around age six months, the frontal lobes first kick in and cognition begins. Between the infant's first birthday and around 18 months, the language areas in the frontal lobes become active. The area towards the front of the left-hand side of the brain is involved with the production of language in a zone called Broca's area. This region produces speech, and was first described by Pierre Broca (1824–1880) at the end of the nineteenth century and in response to studying neurological patients who had difficulty with speech production following a stroke. The pattern of language difficulty he described is called **Broca's aphasia** and I discuss aphasic disorders further elsewhere (see Chapter 4).

Language comprehension is also processed in the left hemisphere, located in Wernicke's area, a zone identified by Carl Wernicke (1848–1905), also in the nineteenth century (Temple 1999), based on observing language impediments in patients that had neurological damage that affected their understanding. **Wernicke's area**, the area that confers understanding, matures before Broca's area; thus for a period of time the child can understand more than it can say, which results in a period of frustration, tantrums and again offers another variable in the 'terrible twos' phase discussed earlier. The science here can be overlaid onto Vygotsky's (1978) theory outlined above, where around this 'pruning' stage his model of language and thought suggests both are beginning to converge to facilitate understanding.

It should by now have become apparent that an understanding of development from a broad spectrum, and one that takes account of theoretical, social and biological dimensions, informs those who are dealing with the normal, and not so normal, pathways that developmentally a child is likely to follow. Additionally, such knowledge can serve to signpost where the child deviates or takes a divergent path from the expected development route.

The importance of early years reviews and screening protocols and surveillance points as advocated through preventative health programmes in England and Wales are discussed further below, and its importance, particularly in early years cannot be overstated.

Activity 2.3: SAQs

- What is a neuron?
- What do neuroscientists study?
- What are the three main parts of the brain?
- Where is Broca's area located and what is its function?
- What role does myelination play in brain development?
- What is the limbic system also known as? Name three functions it supports.
- What is Wernicke's area, where is it located in the brain and what are its functions?
- The thick band of fibres that separate the cerebral hemispheres is called what?
- Where is the motor cortex located?
- Describe one theory about the phase of development often termed the 'terrible twos'.

Reviews, screening, surveillance and assessment

The terms screening and surveillance, often used interchangeably, are related but different activities that describe quite distinct functions involved in the detection of impairments to healthy child development. In the universal health system that operates in England, developmental reviews, screening and surveillance points form an integral part of infant monitoring from pre-birth. This provides ongoing observation opportunities advocated in the preventive programme laid down in the HCP (DH 2009), and establishes protocols for monitoring infant health, growth and development. The review schedule targets health promotion, immunization, and parent/caregiver support. Screening tests are also recommended to 'promote and protect the health and wellbeing of children, pre-birth to adulthood' (ibid.: 7). Concepts of developmental screening and surveillance are defined here but the term 'assessment' is given more attention in the following chapter when looking at disorders that deviate from expected or normal developmental patterns. I discuss this here in broader terms.

Definitions

Screening involves the prospective identification of an unrecognized disorder in development through the application of specific tests or examinations. Specific examination and tests used in screening are not intended to be diagnostic but identify, or eliminate, individuals in a population who are likely to have a particular condition or disorder (Baird et al. 2001). The World Health Organization (WHO) suggests that 'screening is an admirable method of combating disease since it should help detect in its early stages and enable it to be treated adequately before it obtains a firm hold on the community' (Wilson and Jungner 1968: 7). In the UK, all existing screening programmes must meet criteria set out by the National Screening Committee (NSC) protecting and managing confidentiality of information and applying a stringent code of ethics.

A screening test may identify, in a given population, children with a specific risk factor, some of which will be found *not* to be at increased risk when investigated further. In such circumstances, the child would be described as 'false positive'. In the same population a child may also be identified as being at an increased risk, but *not* identified by the screening programme. This child would be considered to be 'false negative'. Screening tests that attempt to identify a specific condition, rather than general developmental delay, or the identification of relatively rare disorders, must have *sensitivity* and *specificity*, terms used to evaluate elements of a quantitative clinical test dependent on the cut-off point above or below which the test is positive. The higher the sensitivity, the lower the specificity, and vice versa. The NHS offers pre-birth Foetal Anomaly Screening for all pregnant women in England and screening for Down's syndrome through an ultra-sound scan between 18 and 20 weeks six days, to check for physical abnormalities in the foetus and/or to provide information to help decide whether or not to screen further.

Surveillance is a term often used as a synonym for screening but is different as it represents closer scrutiny, and an ongoing and systematic collection of information over time by an integrated service system and developmentally at certain points (Oberklaid and Efron 2005). In England and Wales, these points provide an opportunity for assessing growth, and/or discussion of social and emotional development with the child's parents and link into the early years services (DH 2009). Surveillance procedures are seen as non-diagnostic, rather they identify those who need further assessment. As the procedures are performed at several points in time, if a child does not meet certain criteria at one or more of these points in time, this would indicate a higher likelihood, but by no means be a certainty, of the child having a particular disorder or condition (Baird *et al.* 2001). This could include health issues (e.g. obesity/malnutrition) and developmental delays and/or disabilities (e.g. autism, dyspraxia).

In the UK following recommendations to move away from a medical model of screening for disorders (Hall and Elliman 2006) greater emphasis has moved towards health promotion, primary intervention for children at risk, and within the HCP (DH 2009) use tools in surveillance checks, such as the Schedule of Growing Skills (SGS II) to assess children requiring progressive or higher risk interventions. I discuss further the importance of identifying and supporting families and providing interventions to the 'at-risk' child with neurological, metabolic or developmental disorders in Chapters 4 and 5.

HVs, school and community nurses, allied health professionals and general practitioners (GPs) are likely to be the first point of contact when parents have concerns and one of the core functions of initiatives such as the HCP is to recognize disability and/or developmental delay as early as possible in the neonate, infant or the child in an early years setting.

The parent's observations should form a valuable part of developmental surveillance through self-reporting and the use of developed parent-completed surveillance tools. Research suggests that parental reports are one of the most effective ways of detecting developmental delay in young children; that such reports are an efficient and effective way of selecting out children who require a more detailed assessment and are methodologically consistent with family-centred approaches to working with parents (Oberklaid and Efron 2005). In the following chapter, I discuss further the value of parent's data in the identification and diagnostic process, and also revisit the topic again elsewhere (see also Chapter 7).

Pregnancy to five years

A screening schedule, as one example of good practice in England, is given in the HCP document (DH 2009) and clinical guidelines on screening are given elsewhere (NICE 2008). The underpinning ethos of pre-birth, or antenatal, screening is that pregnancy is a normal physiological process and, as such, any interventions the mother is offered should be done so because it has been shown to have benefits, and be acceptable, to pregnant women. Summarized examples of such screening could include the following.

Screening for the baby:

- ultrasound for gestational age/foetal abnormalities and anomalies (e.g. screening for Down's syndrome/participation in regional congenital anomaly registers);
- haemoglobinopathy that can provide a diagnosis/warning/elimination of disease.

Screening for the mother:

- gestational diabetes; pre-eclampsia/preterm; placenta praevia;
- chlamydia – a common sexually transmitted disease (STD).

Screening for haemoglobinopathies can be a part of ongoing investigations leading to pre-conception counselling/carrier testing for conditions such as Sickle Cell disease (where prevalence is reported to be above 1.5 cases per 10,000 pregnancies) and/or thalassaemia an inheritable blood disorder (NHS 2008). In anomalies in the foetus, women should be given information by the health professional about the implications of the anomaly, including options such as preparation, intrauterine therapy, treatment, palliative care or termination. Foetal echocardiography should also be offered as part of a routine anomaly-screening scan. Further antenatal screening that may be offered can include among many anomalies:

- serological screening for hepatitis B virus;
- hepatitis C virus;
- human immunodeficiency virus (HIV);
- rubella;
- syphilis; and
- gestational diabetes.

Appropriate surveillance opportunities are given:

- by the 12th week of pregnancy;
- at the neonatal examination;
- at the new baby review (around 14 days old);
- at the baby's 6–8 week examination;
- by the time the child is one year old; and
- between two and two-and-a-half years old.

(DH 2009: 19)

In the course of promoting health and well-being in children, the level of monitoring and subsequent preventive intervention will depend on the circumstances of the family. The links between pregnancy and learning disabilities, for example Foetal Alcohol Spectrum Disorder (FASD) (see Chapter 5) should be a part of antenatal care and education for new mothers, and promoting sensitive parenting is a vital part of a universal health care programme. Antenatal health and lifestyle advice also needs to be offered to those 'at risk' with the option of an intensive home visiting programme by skilled practitioners (e.g. FNP), multi-agency support and life skills training within social networks.

In terms of identifying developmental disorders, 0–5 years is the crucial period for surveillance and screening. Some disorders become more apparent when cognitive or motor/coordination skills fail to be mastered, or are incompletely mastered because of impediment as, for example, with literacy skill acquisition in dyslexia, or development is not in line with other children of a similar age. Other neurodevelopmental, genetic disorders and/or disintegrative disorders (e.g. Rett Syndrome (RS)) may also not present early symptoms or diagnostic criteria such as described in Chapters 4 and 5.

Genetic screening: science, rights and psychosocial issues

The basis of childhood genetic disorders can be due to several factors. An alteration in one gene, a single-gene mutation, multi-factor conditions, variants in genes and the interaction with the environment will all cause an alteration in function or a chromosomal disorder. In turn, this can cause an imbalance or alteration that underpins an abnormal function resulting in a genetic or congenital anomaly or genetic disorder. At the genetic level, certain predispositions to attention deficit hyperactivity disorder (ADHD), dyslexia, dyspraxia and autism are thought to act in combination to increase risk, and those combinations can vary between affected individuals. Several of the same chromosomal regions show linkage to more than one of the disorders and could therefore share elements that act to increase vulnerability to a condition. Lower incidence disorders such as those described in Chapter 5 invariably result from genetic material being corrupted, through random chance, or misfortune, or from an inheritable line of 'at-risk' conditions that render the foetus vulnerable from its inception.

In Chapter 1, I considered the nature or ecological environment as an influence on a child's development. Here I deal first with children who are considered 'at risk' of developing a developmental disorder and add that I am talking in statistical terms. Risk is a term that can be expressed in percentages or odds. Where high-risk indicators are present in a child's history, e.g. a parent or sibling with say, dyslexia or a disorder on the autism spectrum, it increases the odds that the child will present with symptoms. He or she may *not* necessarily, but the chances are greater when compared to a child who has a low-risk profile, e.g. no incidence of any specific disorder present in the family history. When we are assessing risk we do not profess to make predictions about individuals, rather it is about the likelihood of an event occurring in a population of given characteristics.

So, what are genes and in what ways are they implicated in congenital disorders? Simply put, genes are units of information that act in a complex interaction with environmental influences to determine the structure and behaviour of the individual. It can be considered that there is a genetic vulnerability of a heritable developmental condition for the child *if* such a condition has appeared in another member of the family, over time.

Familial or increased risk to relatives can be estimated by family studies. Twin studies are used to estimate the heritability of a disorder, and molecular genetic analyses attempt to identify the specific allele, any one of the alternative forms of a specified gene, that may be responsible for the measured familial and heritability of the phenotype. The *phenotype* refers to the observable physical or biochemical properties of the individual as determined by the individual's genetic makeup, or *genotype*, and environmental influences. In summary, the phenotype depends on which genes are dominant in the child, and the interaction between those genes and the environment.

Different alleles usually have different effects in the phenotype. Briefly, genes are found on chromosomes and each gene has a designated place on every chromosome, called a locus. Not all copies of a gene are identical and alternative forms of a gene, the alleles, can lead to an alternative form of a trait. Alleles are a way of identifying the two members of a gene pair, which produce opposite or contrasting phenotypes.

Populations at risk are obtained through an analytic process that throws up three kinds of information:

- causes of mortality and kinds of morbidity;
- underlying reasons for their occurrence; and
- susceptible segments of the population.

Morbidity in this context is the rate of incidence of a disorder or disease. I use as an example here Down's syndrome in newly born children:

- kind of morbidity = Down's Syndrome;
- underlying cause = defective chromosome;
- population 'at risk' = unborn child of pregnant women over the age of 40 years.

An independent body in the UK, the Human Genetics Commission (HGC), advises the government about new developments in human genetics and how they might impact on the individual, and from pre-conception, and on their families. The HGC provides advice on the social, ethical and legal implications relevant to populations, or advises individuals about pre-conception genetic screening. Their report (NHS Choices 2011) concluded that no specific social, ethical or legal principles would rule out the use of pre-conception genetic testing as a part of a population-wide screening programme. This type of testing determines the DNA of prospective parents before they conceive, in order to assess the risk of their child inheriting a range of hereditary conditions, some of which are presented and discussed later (see Chapters 4 and 5). A number of ethical issues surround genetic testing and those affected need to be educated and fully informed to make informed choices *if* offered screening.

Ethical issues also underpin many a dilemma about treatment costs with funding dilemmas, desirable outcomes and feasibility of cost effectiveness all having to be weighed up and must undoubtedly hold influence on decisions that have to be made. As an advisory body, the HGC is an invaluable source of information for professionals and prospective parents about genetic carrier testing, preconception advice, identification of problems at the embryonic stage and making informed decisions about termination or otherwise that parents may have to face. Genetic issues are implicated in both high- and low-incidence disorders and this dimension is examined further in the aforementioned chapters.

Summary

- Key concepts in two prominent theories from a social constructivist perspective are those of Piaget and Vygotsky. Piaget offers an individualistic model that stresses the child's individual adaptation to the physical world. Processes of social transmission of one generation to another are not taken into account; Vygotsky's term 'cultural mediation' sees knowledge gained, and cognition developed, through social interactions and shared knowledge of the culture wherein individuals are situated.

- Bowlby's attachment theory emphasizes attachment security, an expectation that key people will be available and supportive in times of need. Attachment figures are those who protect from physical and psychological threats. Attachment styles of *secure*, *anxious* and *avoidant* stem from his early theories.

- Adolescence is a crucial period in the shaping of the concept of self. Brain development changes, physical and psychosocial experiences make a contribution towards the shaping of the individual's identity. Bidirectional and reciprocal influences reinforce self-perceptions.

- Erikson's psychosocial life cycle model provides an eight-stage, lifelong development framework that takes account of changes throughout life and the impact of social experience across the whole life cycle. In the nature versus nurture debate, Erikson focused on nurture and experience.

- Brain development from conception corresponds with physical, social and emotional development. Behaviours reflect brain changes as in the 'terrible twos' and 'risk-taking adolescents'. Neuroplasticity describes the brain as not being a static physiological organ. Throughout life the brain can, and does, change.

- Screening and surveillance points are an effective way of promoting and monitoring health and well-being development in the child, observing where development deviates from the expected profile and identifying high-risk or vulnerable families and children.

- Those in the care of the health professional must be assured about trust, and professionals must adhere to an ethical code of behaviour, be discreet, lawful and fit to practise. Professional associations issue ethical guidelines. These support both the professional and the clients.

- Genetics is the science of inheritance. Genes are the building blocks of life and are frequently implicated in congenital developmental disorders. Genetic disorders can be due to gene alteration and/or mutations in single genes. Multiple factors in the environment can cause alteration of function or behaviour, or chromosomal disorders in the developing child.

- Screening and counselling is available pre-conception for those considered 'at risk' of genetic disorder or in pregnancy where 'at-risk' factors are present. Genetic vulnerability of 'at-risk' children or families can be manifest as a result of the interplay between genetic endowment and the developmental environment.

Recommended reading and further resources

For an easy guide to brain anatomy, see www.brainandspine.org.uk/anatomy-brain (accessed 23 June 2013).

Understanding the Brain: The Birth of a Learning Science OECD. Downloaded from www.oecd.org/site/educeri21st/40554190.pdf (accessed 30 December 2013).

For genetic counselling/identifying clients, a useful article is:

Gaff, C. L. (2005) 'Identifying clients who might benefit from genetic services and information', *Nursing Standard*, 20 (1), 49–53.

Chapter 3 Syndromes, diagnoses and classification of disorders

Intended learning outcomes

At the end of this chapter you will better understand

- the changing dynamics of diagnosis and classification of developmental disorders;
- the meaning of psychometric and standardized tests, the difference between open and closed tests and which professionals can administer specific tests or use specific assessment instruments;
- the range of tests and specific instruments that investigate the cognitive processing profile and measure cognitive deficits and skill attainment levels of a child in expressive and receptive language, literacy and numeracy;
- the three principle 'scanning' instruments used in brain imaging, how they work and what information they can show;
- why it is essential to consider linguistic and cultural variations and their specific effect on test performance;
- the imprecise nature of diagnosis and diagnostic practices;
- the concept of co-morbidity and how this can impact on assessment and diagnosis; and
- different social constructivist views of 'disability' and the underpinning principles of the social model disability.

Key words (defined in the text)

Assessment, atypical, co-morbidity, conditions, diagnostic manual, imaging, incidence, neurodiversity, prevalence, psychometric tests, scanning, syndromes.

Introduction

In this chapter first the distinction is made between the prevalence and incidence of disorders to show the significance of these terms in epidemiology, instruments and diagnostic techniques in the field of cognitive functioning, neuroscience and congenital learning disorders. Psychometric tests are examined, and key professionals identified who can administer and interpret findings from such tests. Psychometric and standardized testing procedures are briefly described, and the significance of a closed and open test and the domain-specific tests are examined. The function of professional bodies is described, as are the significance and dynamics of two prominent diagnostic manuals (The *Diagnostic and Statistical Manual of Mental Disorders* (DSM) and The *International Statistical Classification of Diseases and Related Health Problems* (ICD)). To demonstrate how these instruments have evolved, and continue to develop over time, they are given context within social constructionist traditions. This is followed by an outline of imaging techniques, what function they can serve and demystifying the technology to show how three specific techniques work. The role of neuroimaging as a diagnostic tool is discussed and strengths identified as well as some of the limitations; its role in mapping the brain regions described in Chapter 2 is elaborated. Some of the myths about their diagnostic powers are also dispelled. The problems inherent in the diagnosis and presence of co-morbid conditions are discussed. Finally, alternative models of 'difference' rather than 'disabled' that have evolved in more recent times are considered.

Prevalence and incidence

In epidemiology, the terms prevalence and incidence refer to specific dimensions of a given population under study. Epidemiology studies look at the incidence and prevalence of disease/disorder/condition or problem in a given population. Both terms are closely related and commonly used synonymously to refer to measurements of disease or disorder frequency, but each one has a distinct or specific purpose.

The prevalence of a problem is the proportion of a given population that is affected by a disease/disorder at a designated time. It is an appropriate measure for a relatively stable population, for example, investigating chronic, longer-term conditions. Prevalence is distinct from incidence as it is a measure of *all* persons affected by a disease/disorder within a particular time frame, and is usually reported as the total number of cases or persons with a specific condition, expressed as a fraction or percentage of a population per 10,000 or 100,000 people. For example, recent reports estimate the prevalence of autism spectrum conditions in school children in the UK to be 1 per cent.

In contrast, in epidemiology, incidence means the number of new cases of an illness, disease or other health-related event found, within a certain population under study, over a specified period of time. Most commonly a year is used as the period of time for a study. Incidence is usually expressed as a rate, and measuring the incidence rate is useful in understanding how commonly a phenomenon, disorder or problem occurs over a time frame. Incidence is often reported or expressed as a ratio, e.g. the number of cases/diseases/disorders is the numerator and the population at risk is the denominator. As such, incidence is concerned more with acute disease/conditions but is also useful to estimate the risk of getting a disease. Incidence rates can also be expressed or categorized by different subsets of a population such as gender, ethnicity or diagnostic category.

Assessment and diagnostic instruments

In Chapter 2, the value of a developmental profile was discussed, as was screening from antenatal, pregnancy and through to age five years with several surveillance points in time as recommended (DH 2009). Early detection of congenital developmental disorders, typically first evident in infancy or early childhood, will initially depend on observed behaviours. Such disorders generally manifest if the child is presenting a widely, or subtly, irregular developmental profile, and/or is not achieving expected developmental milestones.

It has been noted that the parent or caregiver of the child is most commonly the first person to alert professionals to gut feelings that something is amiss (Hall and Elliman 2006) and their concerns should always be taken seriously. Parental concerns for their child's development have been shown to be an accurate indicator of developmental problems, and this being regardless of differences in parent education and/or child-rearing experience (Dworkin 2000; Glascoe 2000). Parents are usually very efficient at detecting something is 'not quite right' although they may not understand the significance of their observations.

In children who have no clear neurological disease, criteria-based assessment, rating scales and behaviour checklists are essentially used to gain clinical insights into deviations from an expected development profile. Many diagnostic instruments depend largely on observed behaviours that can be categorized, and identify where impairment is evident in cognitive, linguistic, processing or executive functions, sensory or motor skill performance. Thus symptoms, or signs, that may present an enigma to the parent, can usually be explained and understood from the child's specific profile, when assessed and interpreted by appropriately trained and qualified clinicians or professionals. I again advise a note of caution though, as claims about performance must be cautiously interpreted, as 'rater-error' when one individual observes and evaluates another can, and does, compromise objective judgement.

It is the role of the professional to not only focus on observed behaviour or functioning, but essentially to also systematically record behaviour and performance of the child, because most of the diagnoses used in psychology and psychiatry are actually descriptions, and not causal explanations. The labels we give such disorders do not actually tell us anything about the cause of the symptoms, features or identified traits that categorized observation and/or checklist records. As such it could be questioned: are behaviourally defined developmental conditions, categorical diseases or disorders distinct from normal functioning? But what sets the developmental disorders apart from normal variations in behaviour, learning abilities and mental states is that such disorders persistently inhibit normal functioning and impact on the psychosocial and cognitive development of the individual in the longer term or throughout the life cycle.

The diagnosis or aetiology of the child's learning disability is a significant element and carries major implications in terms of congenital dysmorphology, or development and behaviour. It is one thing to make a diagnosis, but another matter entirely reaching an accurate appraisal of the child's intellectual, developmental attainments and capacities. Testing methods and instruments described here broaden the assessment procedure to identify such a range of the child's assessed specific needs.

In addition, diagnostic categories, or disorders, that are the focus in this book, receive ever-increasing scientific scrutiny, and instruments described here that can aid the diagnosis process are continually updated and empirically tested. This process aims to achieve consistent reliability, validity and appropriateness in identifying aetiology, areas needing remediation, or intervention treatment, and furthering an objective understanding of an individual's functioning.

Psychometric tests

Psychometric tests are instruments for assessing individual functioning in specific domains and are usually administered by a psychologist, psychiatrist or other specialist professional, someone who is appropriately trained and qualified to use the test, interpret the results, report on findings, present a profile of strengths and weaknesses and recommend an appropriate course of action or intervention to address areas of weakness. A **closed test** describes an instrument that can *only* be administered by certain professionals specifically trained and qualified. It is 'closed' to those who are ineligible and only available for use by certain professionals, e.g. *Clinical or Educational Psychologist, Paediatrician*. An **open test** is one that is accessible to a wider range of professionals that are trained or competent users of the test in their professional role, e.g. a HV, specialist teacher or counsellor. Such tests can assist in making a diagnosis or identifiying specific needs, e.g. dyslexia, or they can eliminate specific disorders as possible impediments to normal development. The particular tests for investigating developmental disorders will be discussed within each condition presented in the following two chapters, but there follows here an overview of what specific domain or function each psychometric test explores.

Neuropsychological tests

Neuropsychological tests assess cognitive functions linked to areas in the brain such as memory, attention, mental processing speed or visual processing. Such testing can assist in diagnostic procedures to determine aetiology, or cause, of symptoms, and aid the diagnosis process in conditions such as dyslexia, ADHD, dyspraxia, FASD, Williams Syndrome (WS) or disorders on the autism spectrum. A vital component in the learning process is attention, and different facets or types of attention difficulties (e.g. poor short-term memory, weak visual or auditory memory). As such, each area of attention affected or impaired will have different implications, not only for learning but also interventions to address or ameliorate some of the child's difficulties. In the developmental conditions described in the next two chapters, you will see that aspects of memory dysfunction are attributable to key features. The next activity (Activity 3.1) will enable you to become familiar with how impediments in each specific domain manifest as a learning difficulty for the child. Memory is an embracing term for a system or storage and retrieval mechanisms, far too complex to elaborate on, nor is it necessary to do so. Suffice to say here that different forms of learning and memory are served by different memory sub-systems within different locations within the brain.

Activity 3.1: Internet and online search

Mentioned above are 'different facets or types of memory' or classifications of human memory. Using *selective* and *discerning* skills, search the Internet for descriptions of the following types of memory; find what function each specifically serves and which can act together to perform, or enhance, the same function (e.g. episodic and semantic):

- short-term memory;
- working memory (Gathercole and Packiam Alloway 2006);
- auditory memory;
- visual memory;
- episodic memory (Tulving 1983);
- semantic memory (ibid.);
- long-term memory;
- procedural memory;
- declarative memory;
- sensory memory;
- spatial memory;
- the multi-component model of working memory (Baddeley and Hitch 1974).

A neuropsychological test should result in a comprehensive report that highlights the strengths and weaknesses of the child and, where specific memory impairments become apparent, these should be investigated further in order to address difficulties that as a consequence are manifest. A neuropsychological assessment may assist the family in accessing appropriate health, social or educational support to cope with, or assist them to manage, the identified difficulties or impediments to their child's normal development and learning.

General intelligence quotient (IQ) tests

General IQ tests assess ability, or intelligence, and are *not* dependent on prior learning or knowledge; rather, they look at how good an individual is at problem solving and logical thinking. Intelligence testing is a method by which psychologists measure a child's intellectual capabilities. Although not a stand-alone marker of intellect, as a part of a wider assessment it is a good indicator of a child's academic potential (O'Brien 2001). It also ranks a child against a large sample of children of the same age. Most intelligence tests should not only tell what a child's overall level of ability is, but also whether they have strengths or weaknesses in verbal and spatial areas. IQ tests generally have subtests that will give more specific information as to whether the child is having problems with language-based activities or short-term memory of other areas, and will be discussed further in the context of specific conditions in the next two chapters.

Within the psychometric tradition the focus primarily looks for objective measures with which to investigate individual differences in aptitude and/or ability, personality and experience. Intelligence tests then offer a standard against which individuals' intelligence, or underlying cognitive ability, can be measured, with the most familiar product of intelligence testing being the IQ test. In ability tests there is *not* a pass mark, but scores are compared to how others have performed in the past. An average score is expressed as a mean average of 100 and, in children, that score would be expressed across a population of children of the same age. Over 100 implies an IQ of better than average, below 90 implies a less than average performance or lower IQ level. It measures one educational aptitude and usually includes activities that measure verbal- and non-verbal-based reasoning, visual spatial reasoning, problem solving and logic. Some of the common tests in use in the UK are given below.

Intelligence tests

- Stanford-Binet Intelligence Scales.
- Wechsler Adult Intelligence Scales (WAIS).
- Wechsler Intelligence for Children (WISC).
- Wechsler Preschool and Primary Scale of Intelligence (WPPSI).
- Cognitive Abilities Test (CAT).

The edition in use at any given time will show its continuum of revision, the dynamics of the content and reflecting the constantly changing knowledge base that renders such tests empirical (e.g. WISC-III Third Edition 1991; WISC-IV Fourth Edition 2004 [UK]).

A test that provides subtests that measure a child's performance in a range of sub-skills offers greater insight, and tests such as the WISC-IV, with 15 subtests, yields what is termed a full-scale IQ (FSIQ) arrived at through five composite scores in overall cognitive ability, verbal comprehension, perceptual reasoning, processing speed and working memory. Such tests provide crucial detailed information when investigating specific difficulties and its particular relevance is highlighted in the following chapters (see Chapters 4 and 5).

Problem-solving tests: non-verbal tests

Non-verbal tests reduce culture bias and language bias:

- Raven's Advanced Progressive Matrices (R-APM) are designed for people showing above average ability.
- Raven's Standard Progressive Matrices (R-SPM) are problem solving/abstract reasoning tests for ages 8–75.
- Raven's Coloured Progressive Matrices (R-CPM) are for children up to age eight years.

Specific ability or attainment tests measure skills or knowledge that the individual possesses. These tests measure what the individual may have learned and now knows as a result of their learning. Aptitude tests measure potential or natural ability, or aptitude, for certain tasks or activities. Such tests are prospective as they measure what the individual is capable of achieving or potentially learning.

In summary, a psychometric assessment can determine a child's potential for learning and current level of cognitive functioning (IQ), and determine whether there is a difference between a child's ability and their performance, as would be the case in a developmental condition, or whether they are finding it hard to learn because they have lower cognitive skills or IQ.

Psychometric tests are used to assess:

- ability potential;
- general intelligence and ability;
- achievement;
- adaptive behaviour;
- social, emotional behavioural issues; and
- attention.

Specific reasons for testing are:

- learning difficulties or delay;
- failure in skill mastery, e.g. language and/or literacy;
- underachievement – where there is a disparity between a child's perceived ability and his/her performance;
- emotional or behavioural problems;
- communication difficulties;
- increasing understanding of child's specific needs; and
- concerns about attention difficulties.

Standardized tests and raw scores

First the term 'standardized test' can refer to the design of a test. If described as 'standardized', then the contents of the test are the same for everyone who takes that test. When a standardized test is administered, it is done according to certain rules and specifications so that testing conditions are the same for all test takers. The tester does *not* deviate from instructions in the test handbook. Such tests come in many forms, such as standardized interviews, questionnaires or directly administered intelligence tests. Because of this, standardized tests are suitable for testing large groups of people as they are designed to allow for the individual's score to be measured *against* the score of another. The score of the individual, the **raw score**, is the number of correct responses *for that individual* or in the context of a group such as a same-age population. It allows for some comparison to be made that can show performance of the individual against that of others. But there are other factors that are not taken into account, such as how difficult the test was, where one person stands in relation to large numbers of others who have taken the test and the margin of error in the test scores.

Standardization of a test and standardized scores

Second, when a test has been through a standardization process, it has been given to a very large group, selected by, for example, age, gender and/or nationality. It is important when administering a test that it has been standardized with a population in the country where the test is to be given (e.g. a test in the UK should have been standardized with a UK population). Such tests can provide some type of standard score that can help interpret how far a child's score ranges from the average. This enables individuals' scores to be compared with a large, even national representative sample, as well as providing a score that can be readily compared and/or combined with standardized scores from other tests. Standardized scores are more useful than raw scores and are normally used (a) in order to place test taker scores on an understandable scale; (b) so that allowances can be made for the different ages in a cohort or group under study; and (c) so that test scores for more than one test can be compared with each other. The premise then being, if all tests are standardized through the same formula, this will allow for direct comparison of scores across different tests.

To make a raw score explicable it can be converted to a percentage but that on its own does not relate to the average score of a group, or of all those who have taken the test. Test scores then need to be standardized (given a standard score) so that an average score automatically comes as 100, regardless of how difficult the test is, so it is then easy to see whether a test taker is above or below the average *on that test*.

Percentile rank

The percentile rank – sometimes referred to as the **centile** – is the position of the test taker that can be easily compared with those in the standardization sample. The percentile rank of a test taker is defined as the percentage of other test takers in the standardization population who gained a score at *the same level*, *above* or *below that level*. For example, a score at the 25th percentile indicates a standardized score that is as good as, or better than, the standardized scores of 25 per cent of the sample.

Strengths of standardized tests

- Gives individual scores in a group context.
- Facilitates comparison across a group such as a same-age cohort.
- Relatively low cost of administration.
- Objective.
- Quick to grade and score.
- Gives a quantitative measure.

Weaknesses

- May contain embedded cultural bias – test may be difficult for child outside of the culture of the test.
- Does not allow a child to demonstrate his or her reasoning, logic, critical thinking or creativity.
- Does not allow for/take into account any qualitative information about the test taker.
- Test performance can vary according to mood, motivation or fatigue.

It is important that test users always check the date and size of a standardization sample for the test they plan to use. Norms change over time, tests can 'date' and if they were standardized more than 20–30 years ago be inappropriate in modernity. It should also be age appropriate, suited to the age of the child being tested and only ever conducted by appropriately qualified professionals, especially if a test is a 'closed' test.

Standardized tests have a valuable place in any assessment but always err on the side of caution. The scores they yield will only tell a part of the story in any investigation or assessment. To get a full picture of a child's cognitive, psychological or social functioning, and before any judgements are made about a diagnosis, a battery of psychometric tests should be given, and parent and family observations, pre-school or childcare observations and HV/family nurse opinions should all be brought to the assessment. Contributions from *all* who are involved in the care and protection of the child should be given consideration.

The *Diagnostic and Statistical Manual of Mental Disorders*

The *Diagnostic and Statistical Manual of Mental Disorders* (DSM) I describe here is a significant international publication, widely used worldwide by health professionals, consultants and practitioners, psychologists and the international scientific research community. Published by the American Psychiatric Association (APA) and often referred to as the 'bible of psychiatry', this manual categorizes all mental health disorders for adults and children *in the US*. It basically paired every ailment with a checklist of symptoms, several of which were required for a diagnosis to meet the standard set down in this manual. Known causes of disorders, statistical information of gender, age of onset, prognosis and research alluding to treatment approaches are all published within it.

It serves many different purposes, and is used by a range of professionals not only in the US but globally. Since its first publication in 1952, there have been five revisions and a *DSM* has been in continuous use since that first edition. The most widely used version is the fourth edition (*DSM-IV*) dating from 1994, although this version also underwent a 'text revision' (TR) in 2000 (APA 2000) and as a consequence of research and clinical studies with each revision, the criteria range increases. This ever broadening of criteria leads to further revisions, as well as further editions, with the latest edition being the *DSM-5* (APA 2013). The growth, in terms of number of pages alone in this manual, since its inception is shown in Table 3.1 as an indication of how the breadth of the manual has expanded over time.

TABLE **3.1** *DSM* development: number of pages per manual over time

Year of publication	Version	Number of pages	Number of mental disorders
1952	DSM I	130	106
1968	DSM II	182	134
1980	DSM III	490	265
1987	DSM III-R	567	292
1994	DSM IV	886	297
2000	DSM IV-Text Revision-TR	980	365
2013	DSM-5	991	Expansion in the classification system; considerably more disorders

The latest edition of the *DSM* (*DSM-5*) (APA 2013) has moved to a non-axial documentation of diagnosis, with 20 chapters restructured to place disorders by relatedness to one another, by their similarities in disorders, underlying vulnerabilities and symptom characteristics. Diagnostic criteria for each mental disorder offers guidelines for making diagnoses and, as demonstrated over time, the use of such criteria allows agreement between clinicians and investigators. For more than a decade, many professionals throughout the revision process have tried to ensure each revision is seen to be 'a transparent process'. When new editions are compiled, a draft of the proposed new version is made available for public review, and consultation, revisions, field trials and refinements follow.

To demonstrate how changes are fashioned with new editions and criteria/categories re-established, I cite here controversial changes first in the case of Asperger syndrome (AS) and then with the condition ADHD. Up until the *DSM-IV-TR* 2000 version of the manual, AS was a separate disorder (Reference 299.80 *DSM-IV-TR* 2000) from autism. In the *DSM-5* (APA 2013) the syndrome has been eliminated and collapsed, or merged, into a new classification of *autism spectrum disorders* that the clinician rates according to severity of clinical symptoms as severe, moderate or mild.

In ADHD, diagnostic criteria or symptoms in the previous edition of this manual (Reference 314.01 *DSM-IV-TR* 2000) had to be present from the age of seven years. This has changed and, in the *DSM-5*, symptoms must be present by the age of 12. For the inattentive type, or hyperactive/impulsive type, a minimum of six symptoms still apply. The changes are subtle, but it is good to be aware that these documents are not set in stone, and neither are the conditions that they describe.

International classification of diseases (WHO)

Another such manual is the *ICD*. The volume in most current use is the tenth edition (*ICD-10*) and is described as a medical classification and standard diagnostic tool for epidemiology, health management and clinical purposes. It has a far broader remit than the *DSM* as it is used to classify not just mental health disorders, but is also the world's standard tool that allows for the organization and coding of health information that is used for statistics and epidemiology, health care management, prevention and treatment. In total, it helps provide a picture of the general health situation of countries and populations, and its users include physicians, nurses, service providers, researchers, health information managers and policy makers in all member states of the WHO. Additionally it collates information about health situations of population groups, monitoring the incidence and prevalence of diseases and health problems that are recorded by types of health, and vital records including mortality and morbidity data. The original publisher of this manual was the WHO and, as with the *DSM*, it undergoes regular revisions, with the latest edition, the *ICD-11*, due to be published in 2015.

There are 194 member states of the WHO and the 43rd World Health Assembly first endorsed the principle of a manual in 1990. It was developed from 1992 and came into use in WHO member states in 1994. It is used by professionals internationally, although mostly in the UK and Europe, but does share some comparable classifications and criteria to those listed in the *DSM-IV*. The *ICD* is important because it provides a common language for reporting and monitoring diseases and allows the world to compare and share data in a consistent and standard way, between hospitals, regions and countries over periods of time. There are discernible differences between the two manuals cited here however, as exemplified in the attention, behavioural and emotional disorder ADHD. In the *ICD* manual, ADHD does *not* appear as a discrete category, rather it appears under 'hyperkinetic disorders' (*ICD-10*; Chapter V Mental and Behavioural Disorders, F90–98) and the *DSM-IV* criteria have been found to identify a broader group of children than those identified by *ICD-10* (see Tripp *et al.* 1999 for an interesting comparison of correlates of ADHD using *DSM-IV* and *ICD-10* criteria).

Dynamic effect over time

Constructs within each new revision of manuals lead to evolving subtypes of disorders or conditions. Using ADHD as an exemplar, over time three subtypes have evolved; predominantly inattentive (ADHD-PI), predominantly hyperactive impulsive (ADHD-HI) and combined types (ADHD-CT), and with symptom categorization ranging from a broadened criteria range. The developments of such disorders can be mapped over a series of definitions published by the APA in the updates to the *DSM* as well as by revisions of the ICD.

Attention deficit disorder with hyperactivity (ADD-H) was first introduced as a disorder in the *DSM-III* in 1980 and has continued to evolve over time. The WHO definitions of 'hyperkinesis' have similarly evolved since it was first published in the *ICD-9* in 1978. Categorical manuals such as the two described here are not without their critics, and the self-study task in this chapter (Activity 3.2) will direct your attention towards identifying weaknesses in these diagnostic instruments.

What is important is that making a diagnosis generally involves interpreting information from multiple sources. Information from these criteria-based manuals should form only one part of any assessment of a developmental disorder. Sources gathered should include data from psychometric assessment on standardized tests discussed above, plus clinical examination and a familial history of symptoms. But in Chapters 4 and 5, I give the criteria from both manuals as examples of checklists for identifying behaviours associated with specific disorders.

Activity 3.2: SAQs

- What criticisms and/or weaknesses could be directed at using a diagnostic manual to identify a congenital developmental disorder?
- What information would the *DSM-IV* or *ICD-10* give in the first instance?
- What benefits can you identify in a manual such as either of the two described?
- What psychometric tests would be recommended for a child age six years with difficulties mastering spoken language? What physical developmental checks should also be undertaken?
- What questions would you need to ask before using *any* test with a child under the age of ten years?

Diagnostic neuroscience and imaging techniques

In discussion of the developing brain introduced in Chapter 2, I referred briefly to neuroimaging. This rapidly advancing technology in cognitive neuroscience is providing insights into the distinction between what is common to all human brains and what are individual differences. Neuroimaging is widely used in making physiological diagnosis but particular focus here is how it has opened up the brain to scrutiny. The growing body of knowledge in the field of developmental disorders spans from scanning techniques such as: magnetic resonance imaging (MRI), functional magnetic resonance imaging (fMRI) and positron emission tomography (PET). To understand more clearly how these work and what they show, the strengths and some of the limitations of these technologies are briefly described here.

MRI scanning offers a technique for examining morphology, surveying and evaluating internal structures, tissue and organs in the body, without invasive surgery, or waiting until after death for an autopsy. This technology involves a non-invasive scan of the body, or region of the body under investigation, with the use of magnets. The individual is required to lie in a strong magnetic field and radio frequency waves are directed at the body. This affects the body's atoms, and forces the nuclei into different positions. Most of the human body is made up of water molecules, which consist of hydrogen and oxygen atoms. At the centre of the hydrogen atom is a tiny particle, a proton, and these are very sensitive to magnetic fields. By changing the timing of radio wave impulses, information is accessed that clearly delineates different types of tissue and results in a detailed map of structures and tissue types present in the part of body being scanned. This also presents information from different angles, and can detect defects that may have been present, and building up, since an individual's birth.

The technique fMRI examines anatomical correlates of specific functions and expands the basic anatomical picture that the MRI maps out. With brain scanning it can measure and examine the area of the greatest activity. A popular imaging tool, fMRI is a spectroscopic technique used by scientists to produce high-quality images of, for example, neural 'firing' in the brain. This is fuelled by glucose and oxygen that are carried by the blood and, when an area of the brain is being scanned while a function is being carried out, an engaged location is 'fired up', as these substances flow towards it. The fMRI image will show up an area where there is the most oxygen. The signal transmitted from the firing is then converted by sophisticated software that translates the information into three-dimensional pictures of the region being scanned. Very fast brain reaction to stimuli is caught in rapid frames or images every second and such techniques can therefore show the ebb and flow of activity in different parts of the brain as it reacts to stimuli or undertakes a specific task. Its value as a tool for clinicians and researchers is enormous and, increasingly, fMRI scanning is being used to determine activity for mental processes such as perception, attention and language.

Processes involved are non-invasive, show functions being performed and where disease and dysfunction are present. Imaging offers a localized focus of regions involved in such things as spatial memory functions and effects of disorders such as ADHD, autism spectrum disorder (ASD) and dyslexia. It is also contributing to the growing body of knowledge about developments in molecular genetics, thus helping to dramatically further our understanding of how anatomical systems work.

PET scanning is a diagnostic instrument within the branch of nuclear medicine and uses radiation to produce three-dimensional colour images. The technique is used for diagnosis, tracking the development of a disease and monitoring ongoing treatment, and is also producing a body of research that studies PDDs such as autism. A radioactive tracer is tagged to a natural chemical such as glucose or water and then inserted into the body. This radiotracer will then go to areas in the body that use the natural chemical, and a PET scan will detect the energy emitted by positively charged particles or positrons as the radiotracer breaks down in the body. The resultant images generated can reveal how parts of the body function, by the way it breaks down the radiotracer and produces an image that displays different levels of positively charged electrons, or positrons, according to brightness and colour. On brain scanning specifically, it can show the areas involved in a given task by measuring the fuel consumed, or the areas working the hardest, by measuring the fuel intake in that area.

Fundamentally, neurophysiological functions and structures can be observed through such metaphorical windows that imaging technology provides, but it is a relatively new and developing science. Technology is not infallible. Each method carries with it issues that are best understood in terms of their specific application. Interpretation of the images requires a high level of expertise. Where brain imaging is applied in research that investigates affective components or characteristics of a specific neurodevelopmental disorder, always look carefully at the claims that are being made. Was the study backed up by scientifically valid research? Has the study been replicated to reach a consensus and to what population do the claims apply? While valuable insights are already available, it is an evolving and expensive science and we are a long way from using this as a routine diagnostic instrument. Much more work is needed before scans will be used to make a diagnosis of most congenital disorders, or be able to confidently state that such techniques can identify subtle differences in the brain of a child with, for example, ADHD or autism (OECD-CERI 2002).

Together with clinicians, the scientific community is also making a growing contribution in molecular genetics, as well as furthering our understanding of how systems work. There are neuromyths, or false facts, of which the discerning professional should be aware (OECD-CERI 2002; Goswami 2004) but having said that, studies have shown, and are continuing to show, connections and implicate regions of the brain associated with developmental disorders (Paloyells *et al.* 2007; Ecker *et al.* 2012). Such data will undoubtedly continue to inform practitioners further in their effort to support, or refute, earlier findings, or to strive for even more accurate diagnoses (Stevenson and Kellett 2010).

But I give here a particular example of where the application of neuro-anatomical imaging has begun to make inroads with one particular condition, developmental dyslexia (DD). Images have shown the localizations of the processes responsible for the signs and symptoms of dyslexia (Zeffiro and Eden 2000); and studies have been undertaken that have looked at specific activity in dyslexic and non-dyslexic brains (Galaburda *et al.* 1985; Livingstone *et al.* 1991; Eden *et al.* 1996); and cortical areas involved in reading, object naming and verbal working memory have revealed subtle differences between dyslexic and non-dyslexic controls on tasks that involve specific domains in the brain.

A study with adults with a lifelong history of dyslexia found left-hemisphere regions engaged by normal readers activated in dyslexics after receiving an intervention programme, and that correlated with both their improved reading performance and phonological awareness. Neural activity associated with improved reading also suggested a compensatory engagement of areas in the right hemisphere, and this yielded strong information about physiological changes that correlate with reading skill improvements. The research findings also allow for us to hypothesize about mechanisms of plasticity for later reading acquisition and thus further knowledge of behavioural brain plasticity *even* in the adult brain (Eden *et al.* 2004). Brain studies have also reported that physiological activity changes can be linked to external stimulation and, as such, offer significant implication in a learning context. Scanning techniques have also demonstrated not only the involvement of known language areas, such as Broca and Wernicke areas, but also the contribution of visual pathways and visual motion also involved in reading (Robertson 2000).

In summary, the evidence that neuroimaging is accruing is endorsing the observations of both practitioners and researchers. This technology is a diagnostic instrument that can reveal the complex interplay between developing structural brain changes. Through these techniques, regions have been identified that are engaged in specific cognitive processes, and spatial congruence, or harmony, of the cortical areas, where neurons share certain distinguishing functions, has confirmed the brain's plasticity. Although I cannot overstate the contribution this technology is making to the advancement of neuroscience research, which is where the major benefits currently lie, we are a long way from it being a first line diagnostic instrument for any developmental disorder.

To conclude, developmental disorders vary widely from child to child, and making a diagnosis can be difficult. Conditions such as AS are often diagnosed later in children than a condition where pre-natal diagnosis can be made through an amniocentesis test, blood or gene pathology pre-birth, and is also physically apparent post-natal. While some parents may be aware that something 'isn't quite right' developmentally they may also see a formal diagnosis as an unhelpful label. For others, it can help them to better understand and manage specific needs and behaviours. In terms of a diagnostic assessment though, there may also be an added complication when a child may present with symptoms, or features, of more than one specific disorder. Co-morbidity, or co-existence of, for example, ADHD with dyspraxia or developmental coordination disorder (DCD) has been found to be high (Kadesjö and Gillberg 2001), as has co-morbidity of dyslexia with several disorders such as ADHD and dyspraxia (Pauc 2005), and this I touch on in a broader context in the following chapters.

Reframing disability: an alternative view?

In Chapter 1, the social model of disability was introduced. This views disability as being caused by the barriers that exist within a society, or societal structures, and organizations that discriminate against, or exclude, those people with physical or sensory, mental or motor impairments. In Bronfenbrenner's model (1979), it is within the *macrosystem* that such concepts evolve; the overarching system where cultural beliefs, institutional policies, laws and values are determined. Models of disability can be seen as providing a framework within that system, a frame of reference for society through which laws, regulations and structures are developed, that impacts on the lives of those with disabilities, their families, community or wider populations. For the policy makers, it should go further than beyond changing our language or terminology.

The social model is underpinned with the notion of inclusiveness, including and valuing *all* society's members, giving disability equality and adapting the environment to accommodate or include all. The social model of disability should affect the design and development of services, care, access and the environment, and be written within all policies, but *not* just be passive words in institutional policy documentation.

Activity 3.3: Reflective practice

In your own practice, and on a daily basis, how many policy documents are in place that impact on your daily professional practice?

First, make a list of the ones you think you know about, and what they govern or direct you to do. Then move into looking at policies you are aware of, have heard of, but are not sure of the explicit or implicit directions they lay down for you to adopt or incorporate in your designated daily professional duties.

More recently, concepts have advanced the idea that labels such as 'disability' have negative connotations, and terms such as 'neurodiversity' and 'atypical' offer a shift of emphasis that, it is argued, gives the concept of 'difference' a legitimate platform, in society's terms, from which to view atypical development, as in the autism spectrum disorders, or to account for individual neurological differences. The psychologist and author Thomas Armstrong argues that it is time to revisit our cultural perceptions of disabilities, and that with the new understanding we have of neuropsychological disorders in modernity, we should acknowledge instead the positive differences that a term 'neurodiversity' describes. He argues the point, quite convincingly, for society to consider such a label that allows for people to be seen in terms of their strengths as well as their weaknesses (Armstrong 2011).

Diverse abilities and intuitive strengths such as creative, visual thinkers, or entrepreneurial strengths where 'risk-taking' is often a pre-requisite for success could thus be recognized. As a concept, neurodiversity could be an attractive currency that could just perhaps re-shape society's perception of 'disability'. Certainly anyone who saw the diverse range of abilities, strengths, talents and achievement in the London Paralympics in 2012 would agree that the 'disability' label did little to describe many of the athletes and competitors from a vast international field that excelled there.

To bring to a close this overview of some assessment instruments, I stress the point that to ensure an accurate diagnosis is made, it is very necessary to consider all aspects of development. Always ensure that attention does not solely focus on the primary presenting features of a disorder, e.g. behaviour as in ADHD. Be aware too that diagnosis leads to labels that can, and do, bring both negative and positive consequences for those who are given that label, or have to live with those who have them. I stress also the value of frontline service providers, HVs, family and community nurses and professionals in identifying as early as possible, and following up enquiry into, developmental anomalies.

The two chapters that follow are dedicated to describing features and processes involved in making a diagnosis of specific developmental disorders.

Summary

- Psychometric tests aid the compilation of evidence from which a profile of the child's cognitive strengths and weaknesses become apparent. Professionals involved in any assessment are advised to use instruments drawn from diverse sources.
- Instruments differ in format and will yield raw scores, a standardized and percentile score, or comparative scores from norm-referenced samples.
- A standardized test is administered and scored in a consistent way. The consistency allows for a relatively reliable outcome across all who take the test and can generate quantitative data.
- Most well known of the psychometric tests is the IQ test. Be quite sure of what this test is measuring, it is *not* looking at prior knowledge or learning. It is looking at how problems are solved or how the test taker is thinking.
- Only appropriately qualified professionals can administer *closed tests*, a wider range of professionals can administer *open tests*.
- Diagnostic instruments in neuroscience include scanning and imaging technology; both inform about physiology and organs in the body and measure neurological activity when the individual being scanned performs certain tasks.
- It is not enough for a professional to know the criteria for making a diagnosis in disorders such as dyslexia, dyspraxia and ADHD; many conditions have similar, or even share, symptoms or characteristics.
- When a condition such as ADHD is co-morbid with a condition such as dyslexia, teasing out the behaviours associated with each disorder requires a skilful assessment.
- In the tradition of social construction theory, one explanation as to why prevalence of certain developmental conditions can change over time may be due, in part, to the expansion of criteria with each revision of manuals or tests, or changing definitions.
- Memory is an umbrella term for a set of sub-systems and each performs a specific role as a component of the memory process. It is a multi-system of storing information, for immediate (short-term or working memory) or for future (long-term memory) reference. Knowing the brain anatomy is relevant to gaining a better understanding of how the human memory works.
- The important role of the *cerebellum* is not only in the processing of some memories but also in balance and motor control.
- The *cerebral cortex* of the brain is divided into four major lobes, and plays the key role in memory, perceptual awareness and attention. The *pre-frontal cortex* plays an important role in processing short-term memories and retaining longer-term memories.
- The *parietal lobe* is involved in integrating sensory information from various senses; the *temporal lobe* utilizes sensory information, processes visual and semantic information, and is a key player in long-term memory.
- The *medial temporal lobe* is thought to be involved in the declarative and episodic memory.
- Scanning and neuroscience has informed and validated some hypotheses over time, and refuted other ideas that we held about memory.

- An alternative view of disability can be promoted with less negative terminology. **Atypical** behaviour or development is a term that is being adopted to describe observable deviations from typical or normally expected development.
- In developmental disorders, it is crucial that assessment is objective, broad and takes account of all areas of the child's developmental background and history.
- The social model of bio-ecological systems can facilitate the identification of areas in the child's environment that may place the child in the 'at-risk' category; these may be social, emotional, political or economic impediments, and not even require the child's presence to make an impact or impose barriers to opportunity for the child.

Recommended reading and further resources

For a discussion on IQ tests, their use and interesting definitions of 'learning disability', the following article is recommended. O'Brien describes the shortcoming of IQ testing but also how effectively results can be used according to the purpose the test was administered for.

O'Brien, G. (2001). 'Defining learning disability: what place does intelligence testing have now?', *Developmental Medicine and Child Neurology*, 43, 570–573.

For an overview of neurodiversity as a concept the following reference is recommended.

Armstrong, T. (2011). *Neurodiversity: Discovering the Extraordinary Gifts of Autism, ADHD, Dyslexia and Other Brain Differences*. Philadelphia, Da Capo Press.

Pathways to further information

Equality website, see www.equalityhumanrights.com (accessed 23 June 2013).

The NMC website is an excellent starting point for looking at policies and standards, codes of practice and principles that underpin all community public health nurses and HVs. See www.nmc-uk.org/Publications/Standards (accessed 23 June 2013).

Part 2

Identifying and understanding disorders

Intended learning outcomes

At the end of the two following chapters you will

- understand the difference between low-incidence and high-incidence developmental disorders;
- be aware of, and understand, key atypical developmental signs (e.g. language developmental delay, literacy delay, coordination immaturity);
- know what to look for in terms of features present that can be attributed to each disorder and recognize a profile of features for each one described here;
- know which support groups in the community are a valuable source of further information and where you can advise parents to seek further information;
- be able to objectively support, from a theoretical and informed stance, the existence of specific disorders and/or conditions by referring to, and acknowledging, prominent scientific theories of causality;
- maximize the potential of the Internet and develop appropriate skills to select salient, reliable information about assessment, diagnosis and family support groups;
- have knowledge of the NHS, DH and NICE in order to direct parents/caregivers who are seeking more information; and
- be able to present a balanced presentation to colleagues that addresses the key issues associated with a) higher-incidence conditions and b) lower-incidence, more complex developmental disorders.

Introduction

In Part 1, the dynamics of effecting social change were introduced (Chapter 1); theories of normal social, psychosocial and biophysical developmental patterns were described. Assessment and diagnostic tools through which to examine *atypical* development were also presented. Prominent models of *typical* development were considered, key developmental surveillance points discussed and ethical issues inherent in making a diagnosis, or giving a label, were raised (Chapter 2). In Chapter 3, subtleties were highlighted in the ever-changing diagnostic criteria, and investigative instruments such as diagnostic manuals, that give a qualitative, checklist description of impairments, were discussed. The distinction was made between the concepts of prevalence and incidence, terms often misunderstood or misrepresented in the consideration of epidemiological issues. An alternative view of disability that projects a positive image and supports the social model of disability was also given.

Part 2 of this book is a reference source, a guide to developmental conditions and disorders. These two chapters are structured to give a basic understanding of specific difference observed in high- (Chapter 4) and low- (Chapter 5) incidence developmental conditions. At the end of these two chapters, there is a directed SAQs activity (Activity 5.1) and further research is recommended, signposted through websites and recommended reading. I return elsewhere to examine further interventions for developmental disorders such as described here (Chapter 8) when alternative, and sometimes controversial, therapies, the vulnerability of parents and professional guidance and advice are also discussed.

For each condition a trajectory is given that describes each of the following:

- brief historical perspective;
- aetiology – causal factors of the disorder;
- profile of features – a pattern of characteristic features of the disorder;
- atypical behavioural, cognitive and psychosocial functioning;
- prominent theories and research; and
- diagnostic assessment procedures and appropriate and/or alternative interventions.

Chapter 4 begins with descriptions of developmental disorders that manifest problems with acquiring speech and language (SL) skills, and includes reading and writing (pp. 74–83). First aphasia or dysphasia, terms often used interchangeably, are discussed. European health professionals more frequently use the term 'dysphasia' while in North America the term 'aphasia' is more commonly preferred. Both terms refer to language disorders that can be developmental or acquired as a result of progressive neurological conditions (e.g. Alzheimer's disease), a stroke, traumatic brain injury or a brain tumour. Whether developmental or acquired, dysphasic impediments affect the language areas of the brain described in the previous chapter. The focus of the second half of the chapter (pp. 84–93) is on disorders that manifest sensorimotor coordination, behaviour and attention difficulties. It is important to note here that the organization of this chapter does *not* imply that there is a neat dividing line between the two groups described. Developmental disorders unfortunately fail to have distinct boundaries, and where the child has more than one condition present, or two co-morbid conditions, the problems of diagnosis become compounded and present a challenge to the clinician or practitioner when trying to make sense of a pattern of difficulties that the child may present with.

Developmental disorders presented in Chapter 5, unlike the high-incidence conditions described here, feature pervasive, neurodevelopmental disorders that, in general, occur less frequently in childhood populations. However, I stress here that with advances in science and medicine, more disorders are being diagnosed and 'low incidence' in no way suggests that the conditions described in this chapter are rarely seen. Recognized behaviours, effective intervention and treatment programmes are given for each disorder.

In these two chapters, links are made to further information or support, e.g. further reading, research papers, NICE advice guidelines, family support groups, charities (e.g. NAS, ASF), journals, books and Internet sites/online resources.

Chapter 4   Higher incidence developmental disorders

> ### Key words (defined in the text)
>
> Aphasia, automaticity, automatization, co-morbid, dyscalculia, dysgraphia, dyslexia, dysphasia, dyspraxia, echolalia, expressive language, hyperlexia, pragmatic, receptive language, semantic.

Speech and language developmental disorders

Dysphasic disorders

Here dysphasia is the term used as a generic heading for the focus of congenital, developmental disorders that present specific language and communication problems for children. As a consequence of a specific disorder, language and/or communication skills are not developing as expected for their age.

SLCN in early years development may be transient, or 'not lasting or remaining' (DCSF 2008) and therefore with the right support, the child is likely to catch up and their specific needs will not be permanent. Some children may have SLCN due to problems with production or comprehension of spoken language, with using or processing speech sounds, or with understanding and using language in social contexts. Some may have specific primary SL impairment or impoverished language due to a speech impediment, limited vocabulary and social/environmental restricting circumstances. Or as a consequence of a related problem such as a hearing impairment, an autism spectrum disorder or a physiological problem, causal factors such as weak muscles of the tongue, lips, palate and jaw, with exercise and speech therapy can be strengthened and thus improve the child's articulation.

SL skills develop in childhood in well-defined milestones and parents become concerned if a child's language seems noticeably different from the language of same-age peers. Language 'delay' is a very common developmental problem and refers to language developing in the expected sequence, but at a slower rate. SL impairment however refers to abnormal language development that is very often a symptom of a developmental disorder. The concern in this chapter is the latter, when SLCN are present, persistent *and* a symptom, or indicator, of a specific developmental condition.

Despite their separate diagnostic labels, there are substantial overlaps in practice between dyspraxia, dyslexia, ADHD and disorders on the autism spectrum. But where distinct traits are recognized and attributed to a condition, those differences that set one condition apart from another will be highlighted.

A note of caution

A language disorder that has dysphasic consequences for the child may present as difficulties with expressive language (talking), receptive language (understanding) or both. Some children may show a discrepancy between verbal and non-verbal skills, between receptive and expressive language, or may present with late onset of speech or a qualitative impairment in language and communication development. Others may show abnormal speech patterns including echolalia, where the child presents with an uncontrollable, immediate repetition of words spoken by another person, or reproduces sounds from the environment.

As a child's literacy skills develop, they may present with hyperlexia, the precocious ability to read or decode words far beyond the level of the child's chronological age, without prior training, and importantly, at a level significantly higher than that of his/her reading comprehension levels. This phenomenon will often be evidenced in children with syndromes such as Williams-Beuren or Asperger and disorders on the autism spectrum (see Chapter 5).

Or, if a child struggles to focus on sounds of words, lacks phonological awareness or has an inability to discriminate rhythm, intonations, rhyme or sound patterns, these features too are notable in a dyslexic profile, described later in this chapter. Some children may only have an expressive language disorder, such as difficulties with articulating speech, while in others it may be symptomatic of something that is yet to fully present.

The features outlined here are often features in early years language development of almost any child, but where behaviours described here are persistent it may eventuate as an indicator or symptom of something else. If this turns out to be the case, a diagnosis can only be made when there is sufficient information available to do so. Therefore it is important that *all* incongruities are recorded. Health practitioners and EYFS practitioners thus need to be alert to problems with early language and communication skills that, if left unchecked, could compromise a child's later learning outcomes and achievement.

Recommended publications for further information

Bercow, J. (2008). The Bercow Report: A Review of Services for Children and Young People (0–19) with Speech, Language and Communication Needs. DCSF. Download from http:// dera.ioe.ac.uk/8405/1/7771-dcsf-bercow.pdf (accessed 19 July 2013).

Department for Children, Schools and Families (DCSF) (2008). The Inclusion Development Programme: Supporting Children with Speech, Language and Communication Needs: Guidance for Practitioners in the Early Years Foundation Stage. Archived but available for download at http://webarchive.nationalarchives.gov.uk/20100202100434/http:/ nationalstrategies.standards.dcsf.gov.uk/node/175591 (accessed 2 August 2013).

Semantic Pragmatic Disorder (SPD)

SPD is a communication disorder, where language is used inappropriately or out of context. Semantic information refers to the meaning of words and sentences, and pragmatic information refers to making the language work in the social context. In typically developing children they absorb, process, analyse and then discard unnecessary information, storing the rest in their memory bank to draw on later. Stored information generally relates to feelings, sensations, emotions and basically more abstract concepts. This information can be called on when predicting or understanding the intentions and emotions of others.

The child with SPD has an inefficient information processing system, fails to take account of others and may appear rude or outspoken because of a tendency to speak out, without pausing to consider the reaction to what they are about to say and regardless of any offence they may cause. They may appear to be very good at verbal sentence structure and comprehension at an age-appropriate level, or above. However they have difficulty processing all of the information from a situation, and thus often fail to respond appropriately. They may interpret language literally and have difficulty receiving and interpreting conversational cues. The disorder relates to autism in that it involves difficulties in the three predominant areas of impairment (language, socializing and imagination), the 'triad' of impairment (Wing 1981) but SPD is *not* part of the autism spectrum.

Difficulties

- Using language in a social context.
- Turn taking when talking.

- Keeping conversation momentum going (doesn't 'do' small talk).
- Can be totally unaware of what the other person wants to, or needs to, know.
- Difficulties understanding innuendo, sarcasm, irony and even voice inflexion.
- Fails to take cues from non-verbal language involved in any dyadic situation.
- Problems with abstract concepts (e.g. imagine, guess) or inference.
- Poor social interactional and interpersonal skills – fails to adapt to social situations.
- High state of anxiety when socially floundering.

Main characteristics

- Speaks fluently and may appear more linguistically mature than peers.
- Uses inappropriate language/no eye contact or facial expression.
- Tendency to learn language by rote, rather than the meaning of words; memorizing whole chunks, simply repeating sentences, sometimes with mimic inflection or sometimes in a monotone voice.
- Difficulty giving specific information.
- Can appear rude, arrogant and socially clumsy in interactions.
- Easily distracted.
- Oversensitive to some noises.
- Unable to predict future events, or generalize from past experience or events.
- More interested in themselves than others. Happy with own company.
- Not good at making friends.
- Little or no imagination.
- Temper outbursts.
- No empathy.

Many of these characteristics as you will see in the next chapter feature in the profile of syndromes on the autism spectrum.

Aetiological theories

- Defined as a language disorder in 1983 (Rapin and Allen 1983).
- Neurology, psychology, psychiatric and SL pathology theories.
- A component of other disorders, e.g. AS/high-functioning autism (HFA).
- A separate disorder in its own right but a sub-category of specific language impairment that echoes autistic-like behaviours.

The terminology and definitions cut across disciplines of neurology, psychology, psychiatry and SL pathology all share concerns and debate about SPD, e.g. is it or is it not a part of the autism spectrum?

As the child with SPD is unable to predict future events or recognize similarities in new situations to those that have been experienced in previous situations, they often live in a state of high anxiety. This manifests as a reluctance, or negative response, to change.

Intervention or management of symptoms

- Keep change to a minimum, where it is necessary, give plenty of warning, visual cues and markers towards the new arrangement.

- Teach social skills, using for example augmentative and alternative communication (AAC), supplementing speech or writing for a visual or auditory resource.
- Teach body language, facial expression and non-verbal communication skills.
- Teach different types of sentences, such as *declarative* statements that form a statement (e.g. I went to school this morning); *interrogative* sentences that form questions (e.g. did you go to school this morning?); *imperative* sentences that make a command or a request (e.g. take me to school) and, particularly important, *explanatory* sentences that convey feelings and emotions (e.g. I really enjoy going to school).
- Rehearse given strategies for when the child is over-dominating conversational interactions. Give a positive signal such as lightly touching the child's hand or shoulder. Then when the child fails to respond to signs or signals that a listener is directing at him/her (e.g. looking bored, yawning, looking around) a physical signal can let the child know it's time for someone else to be making a contribution to the interaction.

The management of SPD can follow some of the strategies given later for managing ASD behaviour. Unlike the child with ASD though who will *not* generally react to sarcasm or provocatively teasing language, the child with SPD will generally have problems handling it and become distressed when it is being directed at him/her. The child may also acquire competent directive language, but the tone of the direction can be misunderstood, often received more as a demand and not as a direction (e.g. 'pick that up for me' could be modified into 'could you pick that up for me please?'). Directive language is something that, typically, children usually learn incidentally, through modelling by significant adults in the child's living and learning setting. The child with SPD will not, and will need regularly reinforced teaching to acquire the appropriate use of the directive sentence.

Developmental Verbal Dyspraxia (DVD)

Introduction

Developmental Verbal Dyspraxia (DVD) can be a component of difficulties in the domains of language, coordination, spatial awareness, and movement and motor skills. The motor difficulties of dyspraxia are described in the following section but briefly here I describe DVD or a childhood apraxia of speech.

For reasons not fully understood, the child has great difficulty planning and producing precise, refined and specific movements of the tongue, lips, jaw and palate necessary for intelligible speech. Developmentally speech motor acts become automatic, but in the child with DVD this automaticity is not achieved. Automatization is the process of learning after continual practice, so that the skill eventually operates without the need for conscious control. It appears again in a particular cognitive theory of dyslexia and can refer to learning an automatic response in any skill, whether cognitive or motor.

The HV, in accordance with HCP recommended surveillance points, is most likely to be the professional that undertakes the developmental assessment of a child under the age of three years and thus most likely to be the key professional to notice where milestones are not being achieved. The child with DVD will have presented some, or all, of the following difficulties post-natal, and present with language delay at milestone health checks.

Post-natal difficulties

- Poor feeder; feeding problems usually from birth.
- Poor 'sucking reflex' frequently leads to abandoning breast feeding.
- Major difficulties when weaning from milk to solids; chokes on lumpy food.
- Problems coordinating the tongue; will cope with food pureed; or eat snack food that will dissolve easily in the mouth such as crisps or rice snacks.

Characteristics and difficulties

- There may be a family history of delayed development of speech (e.g. sibling/ parent).
- Problems with articulation, difficult to coordinate speech apparatus, lips, tongue, soft palate, larynx and jaw. Difficulty sequencing the voluntary movements of the oral cavity apparatus to produce or form whole words.
- Difficulty producing sounds, difficult to understand speech; late developing single word vocabulary; early speech is very difficult to understand often highly unintelligible.
- Problems with a limited range of consonant and vowel sounds, difficulty making and coordinating precise movements the mouth needs to make in order to produce clear speech.
- May use a complex gesture system to aid their communication skills.
- Overuses certain sounds and distorted vowels; shows inconsistent speech patterns.
- May have a stammer or reluctance to speak to others than close family members.
- Difficulty sequencing sounds in words, sounding out syllables, using stress or intonation; simplifies words, e.g. 'bur' for 'butter, 'din' for 'drink'.
- Difficulty moving mouth, lips and tongue for eating.
- Sometimes there is also evidence of problems with fine and gross motor coordination – awkward dexterity.

Making a diagnosis

- It is not possible to provide a diagnosis for a child under two years of age.
- Be clear about the home language of the child and the family environment. Could the problem stem from the home setting?
- If any, or most, of the characteristics from post-natal history continue to present problems between 12 months and three years of age *and* speech is not becoming fluent or intelligible, the child should be referred to the GP to start the assessment process/referral route to a speech therapist.
- Usually diagnosis is made by speech and language therapist (SLT)/paediatrician and/or occupational therapist.
- Hearing loss or hearing impediment is always the first area that should be checked by an audiologist.
- Oral structures and the oral cavity need to be examined for any impediment or tongue tie; muscle strength and muscle tone also needs to be examined.
- Diagnosis may be made through assessment by more than one health professional.

Treatment: early prevention

First, parents should be encouraged to keep a record of their concerns and to be specific. They may also have to be assertive about getting a referral for SL evaluation as this service, depending on geographic location in the UK, can have lengthy waiting lists for consultation (Bercow 2008). SL delay can cause anxiety and frustration both in the child and in the parent. In later chapters, the importance of reciprocity in the early infant–mother interaction (Douglas and Brennan 2004) is discussed (Chapter 8) but fundamentally surveillance and monitoring through health visitor (HV) or FNP involvement with parents and families should:

- promote and encourage engagement through language between parent(s) and infant;
- always encourage mother/parents to start talking to their child from birth, or even before, and respond to early babble sounds in a reciprocal, turn-taking way;
- assess parent–infant interaction using validated tools (e.g. NCAST Parent Child Interaction (PCI)).

Intervention and management

- Referral for specialist assessment; parents should work with the SLT, follow their guide and any programme they decide is appropriate: regular and direct sessions with SLT.
- Where this persists look for supporting methods of communication, e.g. British Sign Language signing, talking APPS or programmes on the computer; AAC or Assistive Technology (AT).
- Use gestures along with words, talk to the child in a slow, relaxed way.
- Listen to the child, don't rush to fill in the gaps, or presume to know/guess what they are trying to say.

The health professional should work with the parents to gain access to some professional intervention and monitor the child over a period of time. It may be that the problem is one of limited socialization and/or the family background/home environment lacks the stimulation the child should be getting developmentally.

It may be necessary to refer the family for support or involve social services to get some pre-school childcare for the child. Professionals should be guided by their own knowledge and experience of child development and language acquisition.

Developmental dyslexia (DD)

Introduction

Dyslexia can be acquired, through brain trauma (e.g. stroke, brain lesion) or developmental, present from birth, so constitutional in origin, neurological and will change as the child develops. DD is the focus here and referred to throughout this book as 'dyslexia'. Dyslexia is pervasive and can present with mild, through to severe symptoms that will impact on learning, particularly literacy skill mastery and personal organization. It has been suggested that in the UK 4 per cent of children will be affected seriously enough to require support at school, and a further 6 per cent (or even more) will show some signs of dyslexia, particularly when it is present in other family members (BDA 2012). The severity of the disorder varies and no two children with dyslexia will present with the same degree of strengths or difficulties.

Brief historical perspective

Known originally as 'word blindness', dyslexia was first described by its pattern of difficulties more than 100 years ago (Miles and Miles 1999). Now knowledge about specific causal neurological and neurocognitive dysfunction has confirmed what brain autopsy research had shown three decades ago (Galaburda *et al.* 1985). One of the most prominent theories is the phonological deficit theory of which there is extant evidence (Rack 1994; Snowling 1998). This identified the inability of the child with dyslexia to accurately map phonemes (sounds) onto their respective grapheme(s) (letter or letter string). Genetic implications have been confirmed and children 'at risk' are those where a close relative has a history of dyslexia (e.g. parent, grandparent or sibling). About 50 genetic markers with 15 brain-expressed genes located on chromosome 6 revealed strong associations between one particular gene, named KIAA00319, and low performance in reading, spelling, orthography and phonology, all areas where dyslexia impacts (Cope *et al.* 2005); while a study by Field *et al.* (2013) found that dyslexia genes with relatively major effects exist, are detectable by linkage analysis despite genetic heterogeneity and show substantial overlapping predisposition with ADHD and autism.

Once a controversial condition with many disputing its very existence, dyslexia has now been irrefutably established as a congenital developmental disorder *and* a recognized condition that is a disability. In the UK, dyslexia constitutes a SEN and is recognized as a disability under SENDA (SENDA 2001) and the Equality Act (HM Government 2010b).

The characteristics in the working definition of dyslexia formulated by the Rose Review (2009: 10) are given as:

- Dyslexia is a learning difficulty that primarily affects the skills involved in accurate and fluent word reading and spelling.
- Characteristic features of dyslexia are difficulties in phonological awareness, verbal memory and verbal processing.
- Dyslexia occurs across the range of intellectual abilities.
- It is best thought of as a continuum, not a distinct category and there are no clear cut-off points.
- Co-occurring difficulties may be seen in aspects of language, motor coordination, mental calculation, concentration and personal organization, but these are not, by themselves, markers of dyslexia.
- A good indication of the severity and persistence of dyslexic difficulties can be gained by examining how the individual responds, or has responded, to well-founded intervention.

Profile of features

- Incomplete or slow acquisition of language skills, speech may be slow to happen.
- Slow and inaccurate word recognition.

- Slower processing speed.
- Poor short-term memory.
- Poor phonological processing: cannot map sounds to symbols, cannot detect rhymes.
- Left–right confusion that persists over time or a lifetime.
- Written language does not match oral language.
- Sequencing of events is 'haphazard'.
- Problems with balance, some problems with spatial awareness.
- Tires easily, loses concentration, weak organization skills.
- Autoimmune system often dips: prone to allergies, e.g. asthma, eczema.
- Affects children of all intellectual abilities from low to high intelligence.

Atypical cognitive functioning in dyslexia

- Slow processing speed for decoding (reading) – slow verbal processing speed.
- Spelling may be bizarre and lack phonetic regulation.
- Fails to make generalizations or develop 'automaticity-automatization deficit theory' (Nicolson and Fawcett 1990).
- Retrieving and using phonological codes, weak phonological awareness and speech production.
- Learning to decode may present challenges; some children may become competent readers; but encoding, spelling difficulties will persist into adulthood.
- Disorganized and forgetful, lacking in concentration.
- Brain imaging shows dysfunction of the left hemisphere language network; more use of the right hemisphere than those without dyslexia.
- Impediment may cross over into numeracy/mathematics – dyscalculia.
- Poor fine motor control may affect handwriting – dysgraphia.

Specific Learning Difficulties (SpLD)

More than one SpLD may be co-morbid with dyslexia and include

- dyspraxia;
- dyscalculia – specific difficulties in acquiring arithmetical skills;
- ADHD;
- dysphasia/SLCN/AS.

Prominent theories and research

- Phonological awareness deficit theory (Rack 1994; Snowling 1998).
- Cerebellar deficit hypotheis – impaired motor reaction times, speed of naming (Nicolson and Fawcett 2001).
- Magnocellular theory; auditory and visual (Stein 2001).
- Brain hemisphere abnormalities (Peterson and Pennington 2012).
- Predisposing candidate genes (DeFries *et al.* 1987; Grigorenko *et al.* 1997; Francks *et al.* 2004).

Strengths

- Ability to see problems 'differently' and often solve them.
- Oral skills can be good; good imagination and storytellers.
- Visual creative talents often good; visual creative thinkers, often accomplished artists, good at visual arts and working in the field of multimedia.
- Lateral reasoning, three-dimensional realization may be stronger than non-dyslexic peers.
- Sometimes very skilled mathematicians.

Assessment and treatment or support

It can be difficult to diagnose young children as the signs may not become apparent until the child has 'failed' to master a skill domain that other peers have taken in their stride. This is usually reading, decoding words, sometimes writing and *always* spelling.

However, it is useful to look for early signs as the developmental pattern in dyslexia follows a familiar sequence of the following:

- delays in language acquisition, misarticulating words particularly multi-syllable words; disorganization, a 'scatty' child;
- sometimes late with milestones, often 'bottom shuffler' rather than crawl;
- unable to retain a sequence of instructions;
- day-dreamer, confused by right and left; and
- sometimes handedness is late developing so may be ambidextrous in some things.

Often parents note seemingly small things that when a diagnosis is eventually made, their 'gut feelings' will click anomalies into place. It is usually when the child transfers to a formal learning situation that difficulties become apparent (e.g. processing language and acquiring literacy skills; handling pencils/paint brushes/scissors, etc).

Assessment procedure

There is no one single test that can identify dyslexia, and there is no cure. It is lifelong but it can be managed and, developmentally, things can, and do, improve. Early diagnosis is the first factor that will affect the prognosis, but the quality and duration of an intervention is also crucial.

Assessment should be undertaken by a psychologist or qualified specialist teacher registered to do assessments, and should:

- include a developmental, medical, behavioural, learning and family history;
- be diagnostic, designed to assess strengths and weaknesses;
- include psychometric tests that are both investigative (qualitative) and standardized (quantitative);
- show a profile or pattern of scores associated with a dyslexic profile (e.g. a pattern of low scores on the Arithmetic, Coding, Information and Digit Span (ACID) sub-test of the Wechsler Scales (WISC) described in Chapter 3;
- give information on cognitive processing; language, memory, auditory and visual processing;

- assess both single word decoding, of both real and nonsense words, reading fluency and accuracy and comprehension when reading text; and
- include a dictated spelling test; look at handedness, written expressive language and handwriting.

It was previously thought that one indicator of dyslexia was if the child's reading ability was found to be lower than expected if their given IQ score was average or above. Experts now doubt though that IQ can be a useful or meaningful indicator of reading potential and the discrepancy model is now largely invalid.

Interventions

- Structured, regular multi-sensory teaching by a trained teacher where the student is encouraged to hear the spoken sounds in words, and link them to the written form.
- Teaching programme that targets phonological awareness, word building and word recognition skills; linked to auditory and visual channels.
- Structured home routines and strong home–school links.
- Appropriate in-school learning support and accommodations (e.g. assistive technology, additional literacy support).
- Develop strengths wherever possible – a healthy self-esteem needs success.

Further information

- The British Dyslexia Association (BDA) will provide parent support, signpost you to advocacy groups and have a link to find qualified psychologists, assessors, teachers/tutors in the UK, at www.bdadyslexia.org.uk (accessed 28 July 2013).
- The Professional Association of Teachers of Students with Specific Learning Difficulties (PATOSS) will offer support and advice, and has an index of qualified assessors and teachers in the UK, at www.patoss-dyslexia.org (accessed 28 July 2013). Information is also available from the NHS Choices website, at www.nhs.uk/conditions/dyslexia/pages/introduction.aspx (accessed 28 July 2013).

Recommended books

Reid, G. (2011). *Dyslexia: A Complete Guide for Parents and Those Who Help Them*. Chichester, Wiley-Blackwell Publications.
Reid, G. (ed.) (2009). *The Routledge Companion to Dyslexia*. Abingdon, Routledge.

There is a wealth of information available about dyslexia but a note of caution! Disability law, interventions and resource material as well as public information, where possible, should be applicable to legal systems, education and teaching practices in the UK and, where necessary (e.g. in law and legislation), a UK country (e.g. England, Wales, Scotland, Northern Ireland). The two sites referenced above offer a good starting place. Additional reading and publications are also signposted from these two sources.

Sensory-motor, behaviour and attention disorders

Attention Deficit Hyperactivity Disorder (ADHD)

ADHD is a neurological disorder common in children and adolescents, characterized by clinically significant symptoms of inattention, impulsivity and hyperactivity that are more frequently displayed, and more severe, than typically observed in individuals at a comparable age and level of development (APA 2000). Characterized by an early onset, usually in the first five years of life (WHO 2011) or before the age of seven years (APA 2000), ADHD is a description, rather than an explanation, of a pervasive and persistent impediment to positive psychosocial functioning.

Brief historical perspective

ADHD has a contentious history with conflicting, and often controversial, views posited about the underlying causes, or even its existence as a disorder. Once perceived as a childhood condition, increasingly evidence is highlighting its existence in adults. A myriad of empirical studies and professional understanding of manifest core behaviours in ADHD has evolved over time and diagnostic labelling has followed. In the past four decades there has been a reported increase worldwide in the recognition or numbers of children and young people being treated (Polanczyk *et al.* 2007) with prevalence rates in the UK believed to be between 3 per cent and 5 per cent. The use of stimulant medications to treat the core symptoms of ADHD began in the US in the 1970s, in Australia in the 1980s and has grown in use in the UK since the early 1990s. Medication is currently widely used as a treatment in the UK but is *not* recommended as a first line of treatment. Theories of ADHD subtypes identified three predominant types: 1) where high levels of both inattention and hyperactivity-impulsivity are present (a combined type (CT)); 2) the predominantly inattentive type (IT); and 3) predominantly hyperactive-impulsive type (HT). However, in the new edition of the *DSM*, the *DSM-5* (APA 2013) subtypes have been collapsed into a broader class of diagnostic features that move away from subtype theories.

More boys tend to be identified than girls however extant research is growing that indicates girls are thought to be under diagnosed, may be represented in the 'mainly inattentive' subtype and present more with internalizing problems and anxiety, particularly in adolescence, than boys (Staller and Faraone 2006). Diagnostic criteria for the condition have evolved as research and neuroscience has furthered our understanding of its distinctive characteristics. However ADHD cannot be de-contextualized from changed parenting styles, family patterns, acceptance of different behaviour, cultural phenomena, exposure to trauma and adverse life circumstances that can all be a part of a child's normal day-to-day developing environment.

Aetiology

Although now better understood, researchers still disagree on the exact causes of ADHD, but consensus supports the view that ADHD *does* exist and bad parenting does *not* cause the condition. There is also agreement that the causes are complex, and as yet not empirically established, but the interplay between genetic, or inherited factors, and the developmental environment are strongly implicated. Factors that have been considered in each of the two domains, biological and environmental, include the following.

Biological factors

- Viral infections pre/post-natal.
- Birth trauma – premature birth/perinatal factors.
- Neurobiological abnormalities – prefrontal cortex/anterior cingulated.
- Perinatal hypoxic – ischemic encephalopathy; cell damage in central nervous system (CNS) from inadequate oxygen during birth.
- Neurobiological factors, e.g. imbalance in neurotransmitters.
- Genetic pre-disposition.

Environmental factors

- Adverse family environment.
- Dysfunctional parenting/weak attachments.
- Exposure to maternal psychopathology/toxins during pregnancy.
- Poor/inadequate diet/food additives.

Profile of features

- Mood shifts more quickly to excitability and agitation than in other children.
- Social clumsiness, inappropriate behaviour in social situations.
- Cannot filter out stimuli, attention is shallow, easily distracted.
- Impulsive, no sense of danger, fails to preview event/outcomes *before* risk taking.
- Overactive, poorly coordinated, often accident prone, disorganized.
- Insatiability never satisfied, 'nags' parents, repeatedly.
- Poor working memory – forgets instructions, task or warnings.
- Difficulties with both time *and* spatial awareness.
- Behaviour problems in specific restraining situation/on applied task activity.
- Co-morbid symptoms of additional disorder(s), e.g. dyspraxia, dyslexia, ASD.
- Deficits in rule governed behaviour.

ADHD subtypes as described in the DSM-IV-TR 2000

Essential and persistent pattern of features for ADHD – mainly inattentive type requires for at least six (or more) of the following characteristics that have persisted for at least six months.

- Fails to give close attention to details or makes careless mistakes.
- Has difficulty sustaining attention.
- Does not appear to listen.
- Struggles to follow through on instructions.
- Has difficulty with organization.
- Avoids or dislikes tasks requiring sustained mental effort.
- Often loses things necessary for tasks.
- Is easily distracted.
- Is forgetful in daily activities.

ADHD mainly hyperactive/impulsive type is said to be a subtype if six (or more) of the following characteristics of hyperactivity-impulsivity (but fewer than six of inattention) have persisted for at least six months.

- Fidgets with hands or feet or squirms in seat.
- Has difficulty remaining seated.
- Runs about or climbs excessively.
- Has difficulty engaging in activities quietly.
- Talks excessively.
- Blurts out answers before question has been completed.
- Has difficulty waiting in turn-taking situations.
- Interrupts, interferes with or intrudes upon others.

ADHD combined type is described if six (or more) symptoms of inattention and six (or more) symptoms of hyperactivity-impulsivity have persisted for at least six months. Consider also that:

- not every child will have all the symptoms of ADHD;
- levels of impairment will vary between individuals;
- ADHD symptoms and severity can change with age;
- symptoms such as hyperactivity-impulsivity may diminish abruptly, or present differently with age; inattention may persist into adulthood;
- for the majority of children with ADHD the disorder will persist into adulthood; and
- poor previewing skills – children may be a danger to themselves or others.

Atypical behaviour, cognitive and psychosocial functioning

Behaviours associated with ADHD are best understood as a response to more specific cognitive difficulties, social or situation and/or family circumstances, such as:

- academic underachievement;
- lack of persistence in activities that require cognitive involvement;
- moves from one activity to another without completing any one;
- disorganized;
- poor eating preferences;
- interrupted sleep patterns;
- confrontational and defiant behaviour;
- excessively active;
- reckless and impulsive, prone to accidents;
- learning difficulties;
- poor social skills – difficulties with interpersonal relationships;
- low self-esteem;
- anxiety;
- social adaptive difficulties; and
- high risk of co-morbidity with another disorder.

Prominent theories and research

- Imbalance of brain's neurotransmitter chemicals (Quist *et al.* 2000).
- Cerebellum dysfunction/cerebellar size/volume (Mackie *et al.* 2007).
- Frontal-lobes dysfunction (Barkley 1997).
- Genetic markers (Bobb *et al.* 2005; Farone and Khan 2006).

- Toxin exposure (Williams and Ross 2007).
- Sensory-motor deficits (Piek and Dyck 2004).
- Food allergies/food additives or colourings/mineral insufficiency/insufficient balance in diet (Feingold 1975).
- Executive function – self-regulation/self-control mechanisms (Barkley 2003).

Diagnostic assessment procedures

ADHD requires a medical diagnosis by a doctor, usually a child or adolescent psychiatrist, paediatrician or paediatric neurologist. The child must meet the diagnostic criteria for ADHD in one of two medical manuals, which detail criteria for diagnosis, either *ICD-10/11* or *DSM-IV/5* (see Chapter 3).

Several checklists and/or guidelines perform well in the recognition of ADHD behaviour and offer professionals an efficient way of collecting data from more than one source in the child's developmental environment *or* screening prior to a diagnosis being made.

- Criteria in the *DSM-IV/5* or *ICD-10/11* must be met for a diagnosis.
- Behaviour must be maladaptive and excessive for the child's age.
- Persistent over time (at least six months).
- Persist across more than one social situation of the child or adolescent (e.g. home/school) and can be assessed as such (e.g. Connors 3 parent/teacher/self-report for adolescents) (Connors 2008).
- Must have onset usually in the first five years of life (*ICD*) before age seven years (*DSM*).
- Be maladaptive and excessive for the child/adolescent's age.
- Must cause significant functional impairment.
- Must have no other explanation such as a mental disorder.

Appropriate and/or reported alternative interventions

- Pharmacological Management of Symptoms (Ritalin/Concerta/Adderall (stimulants) Atomoxetine-Straterra (non-stimulant).
- Elimination and restriction diets/restriction of salicylate acid intake (e.g. Feingold diet).
- Behaviour management programme.
- Family support – Child and Adolescent Mental Health Service (CAMHS).
- Structured parenting programme – e.g. the SA (see Chapter 8).
- Alternative treatments such as:
  - biofeedback techniques;
  - mindfulness meditation technique;
  - homeopathy;
  - craniopathy;
  - acupuncture;
  - massage; and
  - sensory integration therapies.
- Diet supplementation Omega-3/vitamin/minerals.

Multi-discipline input could involve professionals in both assessment and intervention

- Psychologist/Cognitive Behavioural Therapy (CBT)/psychotherapy.
- Speech therapist.
- HV.
- Teachers.
- CAMHS child and family counsellor.
- Dietician.
- Physiotherapist.
- Occupational therapist.

The medication controversy

In the UK policy demands that *only* a child and adolescent psychiatrist can, in the first instance, prescribe stimulant medications for the treatment of ADHD core symptoms. Central stimulants have been found effective in the amelioration of symptoms of inattention, hyperactivity and impulsivity, and also on some of the associated problems of fine motor dysfunction and conduct problems. Once stability of the medication regime is established, following regular medical reviews, the child's GP may presume to manage future, repeat prescriptions. Methylphenidate and dexamphetamine are the two most prominent stimulant medications, and these have been found beneficial on conduct problems, academic performance, achieving compliance in the home and school environments. But it is important to stress that even on medication, some children do not show normal, or acceptable, behaviour. Non-stimulant alternatives include Tricyclic antidepressants and Atomoxetine. For further clinical information go to the NICE website for the following reference:

NICE (2006). *Methylphenidate, Atomoxetine and Dexamfetamine for Attention Deficit Hyperactivity Disorder (ADHD) in Children and Adolescents*, TA 98, NICE technology appraisal guidance, March. Downloaded from www.nice.org.uk/TA98 (accessed 31 December 2013).

Long-term outcomes

If ADHD is recognized and intervention management commences at an early stage, then many of the behavioural, educational and psychosocial difficulties can be addressed and the condition successfully managed. But if left unrecognized, or unmanaged, the prognosis is not good. This I explore further when the psychosocial impact of developmental disorders is discussed in Chapter 6.

Relevant research findings

Raine ADHD Study (2010). *Long term outcomes associated with stimulant medication in the treatment of ADHD in Children*. Government of Western Australia. Department of Health. Downloaded from www.health.wa.gov.au/publications/documents/MICADHD_Raine_ADHD_Study_report_022010.pdf (accessed 28 July 2013).

The Raine Study (2010) is a unique data source, a longitudinal study with the potential for further analysis, of children in Perth, Western Australia. This study monitored children at eight sampling points and raises some interesting points about ADHD and medication. Most striking was the finding that children with a diagnosis of ADHD and medication were ten and a half times *more likely* to be failing school than those diagnosed with ADHD and never medicated.

The Multimodal Treatment of ADHD (MTA) study published in 1999 evaluated the leading treatments for ADHD with nearly 600 children (age 7–9 years) randomly assigned to treatment types. The study and its findings are the most cited in the field of ADHD.

For information about clinical trials and development see www.nhs.uk/conditions/ Attention-deficit-hyperactivity-disorder/Pages/Introduction.aspx (accessed 23 July 2013).

Dyspraxia: Developmental Coordination Disorder (DCD)

Brief history

Earlier in this chapter, the speech disorder DVD was described, but here the emphasis is on inadequate or markedly impaired coordination and motor problems. This condition is frequently co-morbid with dyslexia, ADHD and/or some disorders on the autism spectrum. Frequently referred to in its early stages of recognition as 'clumsy child' syndrome, it was first documented in 1937 as 'congenital maladroitness' by Dr Samuel Orton who later became a leading authority on dyslexia and learning disabilities in the US. But it was the work of Jean Ayres in the 1970s that termed it a disorder of sensory integration (Ayres 1972a). Other names ascribed to the disorder include: specific DCD of motor function (*ICD-10*); developmental awkwardness; sensory-motor dysfunction; minimal brain dysfunction (MBD); and motor sequencing disorder to name but a few. It affects approximately 2 per cent of the population in one degree or another and 70 per cent of those affected are male. Dyspraxia is sometimes called the 'hidden disability' because those affected show no outward signs of being disabled.

Aetiology and prominent theories

- Birth related, e.g. premature birth, low birth weight, birth trauma, mother drinking alcohol/drug taking.
- Acknowledged as being an immaturity of the brain. Connections between groups of neurones may not fully develop resulting in messages not being relayed properly to/from sensory channels in the body.
- Possible damage caused by birth trauma or lack of lipids (fats) in the diet at important post-birth stages.
- Immaturity of physical features of cerebral cortex so there is insufficient control of the limbic system; this shows as difficulty controlling emotions/child overactive.
- Vestibular receptors in the inner ear that sense where the body is in relation to the environment are impaired in dyspraxia.
- Proprioceptive system in the body in some way impaired; child with dyspraxia lacks the sense of placement. Fails to judge where the body is in relation to objects.

Profile of features

Dyspraxia can affect any, or all, areas of development: physical, social, emotional, language and many areas of learning.

Birth to five years

- Feeding, poor breast feeders, doesn't develop sucking reflex.
- Irritable babies, sleep patterns are poor, cries a lot; as an infant, waves arms and legs around vigorously as if falling.
- Messy eater, spills things, late learning to feed her/himself, uses fingers rather than spoon or knife and fork.
- Frequently presents with speech difficulties.
- Late reaching developmental milestones; delays also in non-motor milestones.
- Frequently falls or bumps into things; inability to sit still.
- Takes longer than expected to roll over/sit/crawl/walk.
- Slow to master toilet training.
- Difficulties clasping or grasping for a toy or article at a very early age; poor gross and fine motor skill performance; problems trying to catch a ball/bean bag.
- Poor balance, difficulty and slowness getting dressed, learning to tie laces, do/undo buttons; late learning to dress him/herself; frequently puts clothes on in the wrong order.
- Short attention span; not always successful forming play relationships; poor social skills.

Age 5–19 years

- A particular 'gait' when walking, often holds onto the walls.
- Slow responder; poor problem solvers.
- Difficulty using a knife and fork; or any tool that requires dexterity (e.g. scissors).
- Late learning to ride a bike, use a scooter/balance, hop or skip.
- Poor spatial awareness, timing and rhythm, slow to generalize learned skills.
- Impaired coordinated movement/hand–eye coordination skills; persists in adulthood.
- Poor handwriting; organization, self-management/poor time management.
- Slow to understand abstract concepts, relies on concrete examples longer than peers.
- Poor posture, tends to loll or drape body across desk or tables, frequently sits with a foot underneath them and this lasts into adolescence and beyond.
- Tactile senses may be heightened; poor understanding of sensory information; perception problems.
- Poor gross and fine motor skills persisting into adulthood.
- Difficulties forming and sustaining relationships.
- Academic problems, fails to meet deadlines, doesn't keep up with the group; slow to grasp concepts, organize ideas, get things written down; frequently falls behind peers in skills and knowledge acquisition.

A poor kinaesthetic and proprioceptive sense shows in the child as:

- a poor sense of poise, easily tired by the constant effort to stay erect;
- constantly fidgeting to get feedback to help balance;
- having poor depth perception causing stumbling, tripping or falling over;
- having poor sense of direction.

Making a diagnosis

- Parents should share concerns with HV or GP and ask for a referral to a paediatrician, or a multi-disciplinary team in a child development centre. Parent can also consult the school nurse, community-based team, school doctor or occupational therapist for practical guidance and coping strategies.
- Parent can discuss their concerns with the child's teacher, the SENCO, the school nurse, school doctor or GP.
- A referral request can be made through a paediatrician, hospital or community-based therapy team, educational psychologist or child and family support team.
- A paediatrician will assess and make recommendations of who else is to be involved in the therapy or intervention plan.
- A paediatric occupational therapist.

Further information

The Dyspraxia Foundation, a registered charity, offers support and information to parents and professionals, see www.dyspraxiafoundation.org.uk (accessed 18 July 2013) or www.nhs.uk/Conditions/Dyspraxia-(childhood)/Pages/Introduction.aspx (accessed 18 July 2013).

Recommended books for further information

Kirby, A. (2006). *Dyspraxia: The Hidden Handicap*. London, Souvenir Press (E&A).
McKeown, S. (2012). *How to Help your Dyslexic and Dyspraxic Child: A Practical Guide for Parents*. Surrey, Crimson Publishing.
Portwood, M. (2000). *Understanding Developmental Dyspraxia: A Textbook for Students and Professionals*. London, David Fulton Publishers.

Deficits in Attention, Motor Control and Perceptual Abilities (DAMP)

I have included this disorder for two reasons. First, it is a lesser known disorder, though not necessarily a 'low-incidence' one that warrants inclusion in the following chapter. Second, the concept has been around since the 1970s in Scandinavian countries, as a label that originally operationalized what at that time was called MBD (Gillberg 2003). Its important because clinically it fits somewhere between ADHD plus DCD/dyspraxia. The DAMP construct is then useful for identifying children *with* ADHD or DCD *and* multiple needs that would not be self-evident if a diagnosis is given as *just* ADHD or *just* DCD.

When the features are described, the overlap between DAMP, ADHD and DCD/dyspraxia and developmental disorders described in this and the next chapter become very apparent. But it may be questioned as to whether this is a disorder in its own right or, indeed, if it has something specific that distinguishes it from the rest. Here I support the view expressed by Gillberg (2003) that this construct has an interactive role, as it falls between two distinct and high-profile disorders. Clinically, this allows for a more comprehensive description of what domains are impaired and what diagnostic procedures can help identify impairments. Few of those with a diagnosis of DAMP do well in the longer term without specific help, and this is a valid reason as to why the concept may be helpful in clinical practice.

Brief history

In 1974, Bengt Hagberg, a child neurologist, initiatied a large-scale empirical study of MBD. Other studies followed, out of which the concept of DAMP emerged. The term has been widely used since then in Scandanavian countries, Europe, the UK and Australia; and Gilberg and colleagues have been associated with many empirical research studies worldwide since the 1980s. In Sweden, DAMP pre-dates ADHD as the term was used in Scandinavia prior to the publication of the *DSM-III-R* (1987) where ADHD appeared for the first time.

Aetiology

There is an overlap between various other developmental disorders and DAMP which is a combination of motor control and perceptual problems in addition to problems with attention. Children with DAMP may not have any definite neurological dysfunction or difference in brain structures, but it is thought the networks in the brain behave differently to children that do not have DAMP. DAMP is frequently co-morbid with SL problems, ADHD and/or dyslexia.

Profile of features

- Attention problems, unable to sit still, short concentration span.
- Slow processors; need time to process information or perform executive functions.
- Cordination difficulties; fine and gross motor skills impaired.
- Hypotonia – weak muscle development, reluctance to 'stretch' muscles/extend limbs.
- Clumsiness, lack of balance, spills food and drink easily, messy eating.
- Reluctant to participate in organized sports or physical activities.
- Perceptual difficulties, visual perceptual tasks difficult, drawing, writing and even reading present problems/left–right orientation of reading a difficult concept to grasp; organizing writing on paper is a problem.
- SL problems; articulation of some words.

Atypical behaviours

- Physical developmental delay, difficulties judging distances, body parts in space, spatial awareness problems.
- Perceptual problems can cause falls, collisions and accidents; child accident prone, clumsy, prone to tumbles/tripping/falls.
- Delayed SL development – immature pronunciation of words.

Making a diagnosis

- Detailed developmental history from primary carer and health professional (e.g. HV).
- Rating against a rating scale/criteria scale for ADHD (e.g. *DSM* or *ICD* manuals).
- Neuromotor assessment by a paediatrician.
- Deficits in height/weight/head circumference/vision/hearing and screening for physical development abnormalities using such instruments as SGS II.
- Severe cases should have electroencephalography (EEG) to eliminate cerebral palsy or other cerebral factor as the cause.
- Karyotype test to eliminate gene deletion/genome impairment.
- Very severe cases, MRI scan to look for non-developmental underlying cause/ deteriorating or degeneration causal factors.
- Multi-professional assessment to look for social, educational or developmental needs.

Appropriate intervention

- Occupational and physiotherapy involvement to address motor control dificulties.
- Psycho-educational needs, individual education programme with clearly set, supported targets will help the school-age child with DAMP.
- SLT required in some cases.
- Psychotherapy in adolescence may be considered appropriate to deal with behaviour difficulties and adjustment/conduct disorders that may prevail.
- If attention problems impede learning, or behaviours are difficult to regulate, psychopharmacology, stimulant medication, shown to have a positive effect on ADHD symptoms, may well be successful with the child diagnosed with DAMP *but only as a last resort and after all other treatments have first been explored.*

To conclude, the DAMP concept has had an important, if not momentary, effect in much the same way as the concept of AS had in terms of autism spectrum disorders. It has helped to draw attention to an important sub-group and in as much as some families are more comfortable with a diagnosis of AS for their child then too may some families be more comfortable with DAMP as opposed to ADHD and the many controversial issues that surround this developmental disorder.

Summary

- Physiological and developmental impediments that contribute towards SL delay can be described as dysphasic. Some SLCN are transient and usually categorized as 'language delay'.
- There is an overlap across developmental disorders where symptoms may be present in more than one disorder, including ADHD, DVD and disorders on the autism spectrum. Receptive and expressive language may be affected.
- Two or more disorders may be co-morbid, and symptoms of each difficulty may be difficult to 'tease out'. Food allergies and dietary issues may be present in more than one condition. Feeding and poor sucking reflexes may eventually be identified as a feature of SL anomalies; SL difficulties may be a feature in more than one disorder.

- Understanding the meanings of words may not be complete in SPD, and the child unable to engage in the pragmatics or meaning of language itself. Turn taking, social engagement, taking cues and expression of emotions or feelings are features that are lacking.
- DVD may be underpinned by immature physiological structures of the oral cavity and oral structures including the mouth, jaw, lips and tongue. It may also present as a part of a dyspraxia profile, where motor skill development is compromised.
- Dyslexia is a neurological disorder constitutional in origin, highly heritable and affects the smooth acquisition of the literacy skills of reading, writing and spelling. It will change over time, but is not curable. Most dyslexics learn coping strategies; reading may not be a problem to all of those with dyslexia; spelling is a lifelong problem for *all* dyslexics.
- ADHD is *not* the result of bad parenting, laziness, poor motivation, low intelligence or disobedience. Problems faced by children with ADHD go well beyond the symptoms of inattentiveness, hyperactivity and impulsivity. Treatment should involve medication only as the last line of treatment unless there are exceptional circumstances. A multi-modal model of support should be available for the child.
- ADHD can be managed but is lifelong, can be pervasive and very debilitating affecting daily life functioning, academic performance, behaviour in school, peer relationships, siblings and parents.
- DAMP is a disorder that fits somewhere between ADHD and DCD and presents with the features of both but such features as perception, motor-perceptuo difficulties and impaired performance of executive function skills are also present.

The conditions that have been described in this chapter are all chronic, debilitating and need to be addressed in terms of *any* intervention that will be of value to the diagnosed individual across his or her lifetime.

In Chapter 5 that follows, developmental disorders are presented that also impact on living and learning over a lifetime, as well as the role of the family nurse and/or HV in the assessment and management of such disorders.

Chapter 5   **Lower incidence developmental disorders**

Intended learning outcomes

At the end of this chapter you will

- understand the main characteristics of each developmental disorder described;
- critically review causal models from the literature for each of the described neurological disorders;
- be aware of, and understand, key atypical developmental signs (e.g. language, communication or literacy delay; coordination immaturity);
- understand the inherent difficulties of identification and diagnosis in a developmental disorder;
- know which 'at-risk' biological and social factors would alert the health professional to potential disorders;
- know what key information should be collected and/or acted upon when presented with developmental anomalies in a child; and
- know what to look for in terms of features present and recognize the primary specific profile of features for each disorder.

Key words (defined in the text)

Asperger Syndrome (AS), autism spectrum disorder (ASD), central nervous system (CNS), foetal/fetal, Foetal Alcohol Syndrome (FAS), high-functioning autism (HFA), neurological, Rett Syndrome (RS), salicylates, teratogenic, Williams-Beuren Syndrome (WBS).

Introduction

In an earlier chapter (see Chapter 2) genetic issues in neurodevelopmental disorders were introduced and here a connection is made to conditions within this broad category. The heritability and common phenotype, current thinking on the nature and the key characteristics of each are given.

Many conditions also overlap in terms of impact on neurological functioning developmentally and this will become apparent as neurocognitive deficits and dysfunctions are described here. Disorders that impact on behaviour also share similar traits such as poor attention, genetic or hereditary components and, similarly, theories about cause and effect may implicate the same sensitivities. I briefly mention here an example of one such 'sensitivity', the issue of diet, aligned particularly to attention and behavioural issues.

In the previous chapter, and the chapter that follows, you will note that manifest feeding difficulties in infancy and early years are a feature in more than one developmental condition. Implicated are such issues as food texture, strong tastes or smells, or difficulties with the digestion of certain foods. Food allergies have also been associated with more than one condition, and research has investigated how symptoms may, or may not, respond effectively to elimination diets. Research has also looked for connections to dietary links and developmental conditions through salicylates, chemicals naturally occurring in some foods (Stevens *et al.* 2010); lactose, gluten and casein intolerances (Erickson *et al.* 2005; Elder *et al.* 2006); or exclusionary diets that support or refute anecdotal reports of the benefits (Millward *et al.* 2009).

Supplemented diets too have been explored, notably Omega-3 essential fatty acids (EFA), and linked to favourable outcomes in children with dyspraxia, dyslexia and ADHD (Richardson 2002) as well as disorders that are on the autism spectrum (Amminger *et al.* 2007). The health professional needs to be aware of these issues as programmes often feature 'high-profile' diets that sometimes allegedly 'cure' or ameliorate symptoms and parents will, understandably, be pressing for more information. I return to this issue in Chapter 8 when parent vulnerability is discussed further.

I stress again that due care be given when considering the presence of *any* condition. Many features described here relate to normal developmental features that present in different stages as the child matures. What is different here though is the persistence or worsening of features as the child develops. Also, in all disorders there will be a range of impacting difficulties from those children presenting with some, several or, occasionally, all symptoms. No two children even with the same disorder will present with an identical set of features. As such there is a need for professionals to undertake a multi-faceted assessment before any decision is made that favours the diagnosis of one disorder over another.

Aetiology, or causal theories, age of onset, characteristics and/or manifest behaviours, assessment instruments and diagnostic criteria are given. Features common across conditions that resemble each other, as well as specific features that set each one apart, are acknowledged. Links are given to recommended additional reading and current research. Useful sources of information for family and professional support are also given for each disorder.

Neurological disorders

The specific causes of neurological disorders are various and I include within this broad category genetic disorders, congenital abnormalities, single gene disorders/gene deletion/chromosomal disorders; conditions associated with environmental or life-style problems such as FAS disorders; or, following infection, disease or impoverished diet, chronic health conditions and/or degenerative disorders. I also make the distinction here between a specific disorder and what is more generally coined as a pervasive developmental disorder – not otherwise specified (PDD-NOS).

This generally refers to a child that may present fewer, or less pronounced, characteristics of autism, atypical autism or AS. The child may even be given an autism diagnosis at a later age or developmental stage, but the term itself should direct professionals to explore options for child and family support, appropriate services and even intervention for the child and family concerned.

Foetal Alcohol Syndrome (FAS)/Spectrum Disorder (FASD)

Brief historical perspective

FASD[1] is an umbrella term that describes a range of impacting adverse effects that can occur in an individual, as an effect of pre-natal alcohol exposure or if the mother drank alcohol during pregnancy. The harmful effects of alcohol on the foetus, and the connection between pre-natal alcohol exposures although known about and first publicly reported in 1899 by Dr William Sullivan of Liverpool, first began to appear in the medical and scientific domains in the 1950s and 1960s. Prominent early studies are those of Jacqueline Rouquette in 1957 and a paper by Dr Paul Lemoine in 1968, however, it wasn't until two paediatricians in Seattle, David Smith and Ken Jones, had a paper published in the medical journal *The Lancet* in 1973 that the term 'fetal alcohol syndrome' disorders was first used (www.fasdcenter.samhsa.gov). With increases in binge drinking, particularly in young people, FASDs are a concern both nationally and internationally and information given here comes from a range of international and national public awareness and public health literature referenced below.

Aetiology

Research supports a positive correlate association between excessive consumption of alcohol by women who are pregnant and FASD. FASDs are preventable but once the damage is done it is irreversible. The range of phenotypes associated with FASD will vary in severity and outcome that will depend on the level, pattern and timing of maternal alcohol consumption. Alcohol is a teratogenic compound, a substance that interferes with the normal development of the embryo or foetus, because it crosses the placenta (BMA 2007). The foetus is totally unprotected due to the absence of a developed blood filtration system, thus pre-natal alcohol exposure affects the foetus in many ways. It is during the first eight weeks of embryogenesis that the primary teratogenic effect occurs, while exposure later in the pregnancy may affect growth, behavioural and cognitive disorders.

Incidence and prevalence varies across populations worldwide, but is highly reported in African American groups in the US, indigenous groups in Canada and in Australia, and coloured/mixed races in South Africa. Worldwide factors that appear to increase

97

the risk of FASD occurring are in particular low socio-economic status, pattern of drinking, age or duration of drinking, genetic predisposition, maternal nutrition and health, smoking and loss of traditional culture (O'Leary 2002). In the UK, FASDs are reported as being the most common, non-genetic cause of learning disability, and in Europe affects around 1 per cent of live births (see Blackburn *et al.* 2009).

It cannot be stressed strongly enough that clear guidance must be given to inform pregnant women, or those who are trying for a baby, of the risk factors involved with alcohol consumption. A spectrum of disorders and individual anomalies are embraced within the phenotype FASD that include impaired attention, behavioural and learning disabilities and cognitive development, all of which are lifelong issues. As with all developmental disorders, the profile of features given here are not a prescriptive checklist. Some more than others may be present, while in other infants, all features may be identified depending on the factors given above. The spectrum of syndromes within the umbrella term FASD are:

- **FAS** – a specific identifiable group of children with specific facial features, CNS dysfunction and many of the characteristics given below. These symptoms form only when maternal alcohol consumption occurs during the first trimester, or first three months, of a pregnancy.
- **Partial Foetal Alcohol Syndrome (pFAS)** – from maternal alcohol exposure, child may exhibit some, but not all, physical features of FAS, CNS damage demonstrated through learning and behavioural difficulties developmentally.
- **Alcohol-related Neurodevelopmental Disorder (ARND)** – CNS damage from confirmed history of pre-natal alcohol exposure. Poor impulse control, poor social skills, weak memory and low attention span.
- **Alcohol-related Birth Defects (ARBD)** – physical anomalies related to pre-natal alcohol exposure and can include heart defects; skeletal, vision and hearing problems, fine and gross motor impairments.

The complexity of the disorder may be compounded further by the overlap of co-morbid, or co-existing, conditions such as ADHD, ASD or other developmental disorders. Additionally secondary factors such as the family history, home and life circumstances may present barriers to a positive prognosis for the child, and families affected will most probably require a strong, multi-agency health and social care support programme pre- and post-natal.

Profile of features: a pattern of characteristics

- Significant delays in achieving developmental milestones such as toileting, language development and motor skills.
- Discriminating physical features that include: flat mid-face, short flat nose, low nasal bridge, thin upper lip.
- Growth retardation.
- Pre-natal growth deficiency – small for gestational age.
- Post-natal growth deficiency – lack of catch-up growth despite good nutrition.
- Low weight-to-height ratio.
- Microcephaly or abnormally small head due to failure of brain growth and/or other structural defects.

Atypical behaviour, cognitive and psychological functioning

- CNS anomalies or dysfunction.
- Developmental delay, learning, attention and behavioural disorders.
- Sensory impairments and sensory processing difficulties. Seeking enhanced and continuous sensory inputs (e.g. hyperactivity, distractability, irritability, inattention).
- Intellectual disability.
- Frontal lobe damage in the brain, impaired executive functioning.
- Poor hand–eye coordination, maybe tremors, impaired fine motor control and balance.
- Neurological abnormalities in domains such as communication, memory, visual and spatial skills, motor skills.
- Sleep pattern disturbances, attention deficits, poor visual focus, delayed speech.
- Social and emotional problems that impact on relationships.

Prominent theories and research

The timing and intensity of maternal alcohol exposure, the dose and frequency is generally accepted as the principal determinant of functional deficits (see Clarren *et al.* 1992). Diagnosis is controversial and there is a paucity of knowledge about how best to support children and families affected through education, health and social services. One exception in England is the project undertaken by University College Worcester in 2009–2010. For the research report reference and website where this is available, see Blackburn (2009).

Making a diagnosis

The diagnosis is based on a set of criteria and abnormalities in three main areas: growth retardation, characteristic facial features and CNS anomalies. These include intellectual impairment that is intractable and permanent.

Making a diagnosis usually requires a clinical input from a paediatrician or physician, and how easy or difficult diagnosis is will depend on the features and severity of symptoms presented. If characteristic malformation of the facial features, or dysmorphology, is present, diagnosis may be relatively straightforward; otherwise developmental anomalies need to correlate with observations and mother's pregnancy history. In many cases a paediatrician will have been involved since pre-birth, as mother's pre-natal care should have identified 'at-risk' factors during the pregnancy and other health and care services, early years services and support agencies may also have been alerted before the birth.

Counselling prior to the birth of the child is recommended for the child's parent(s) and screening, monitoring and surveillance scans are recommended to identify the nature of related issues that may be anticipated. A multi-disciplinary approach to managing the child's symptoms and behaviour is recommended, and parents and families affected should be directed through their frontline health professional to a support group and/or support network (e.g. National Organisation for Foetal Alcohol Syndrome (NOFAS) UK).

Appropriate intervention

- Support structures should be put in place pre-natal.
- After first gaining consent from the parent/family to share information, begin to build a team around the child (TAC) as early as possible. The TAC is a holistic approach to support the child and family (see Chapter 9).
- Effective communication links between the family and the health and social care professionals. Use the CAF to gather and collate information in relation to the child's needs in development, parenting and the family environment.
- Using the structures of an Education Healthcare Plan (EHCP) (see Chapter 9) to identify needs, resource provision, review developmental progress and changed needs over time.
- Management of environmental factors through involvement of multi-agencies with a lead professional (e.g. issues such housing, child protection, early years childcare opportunities).
- Pre-school, early years education and school support will be required, the nature of which will be determined by the severity of the child's physical or intellectual development.
- Support provision will need to be ongoing throughout their life and into adulthood.

Further reference sources

- British Medical Association (BMA) Board of Science (2007). *Fetal Alcohol Spectrum Disorders: A Guide for Healthcare Professionals.* London, BMA.
- NOFAS UK. www.nofas-uk.org (accessed 28 July 2013). An excellent framework compiled by Carolyn Blackburn (Oct 2010) free to download and available from this website.
- US Department of Health and Human Services. Substance Abuse and Mental Health Services Administration (SAMHSA) Center for Substance Abuse Prevention. www.fasdcenter.samhsa.gov (accessed 12 May 2013).
- Fetal Alcohol Syndrome: a Literature Review (August 2002). Prepared by Colleen O'Leary. National Alcohol Strategy. Publication 3125. Commonwealth Department of Health and Ageing. Australia. www.health.gov.au/internet/alcohol/publishing.nsf/Content/746BAD892492B586CA2572610010C29A/$File/fetalcsyn.pdf (accessed 31 December 2013).
- Blackburn, C. (2009). Foetal Alcohol Spectrum Disorder: Focus of Strategies. Building Bridges with Understanding Project. Sunfield Research Institute and Worcestershire County Council UK. www.sunfield.org.uk/pdf/FASD_Building_Bridges.pdf (accessed 31 December 2013).

Rett Syndrome (RS)

Brief history

The neurodevelopmental disorder RS is a degenerative disease. Clinically and not genetically defined, this condition should not be dismissed as presenting in boys, but it almost exclusively affects girls (Leonard *et al.* 2001). It was first clinically described relatively recently, in 1966, by the Austrian physician Dr Andreas Rett, and appeared again later, in 1983, in a paper by Swedish researcher Dr Bengt Hagberg. The gene mutation implicated in RS was first identified in 1999 (Amir *et al.* 1999), and in the past two decades, has gained increased worldwide clinical recognition. Advances in epigenetics, the study of heritability, neurobiology and molecular genetics, are collectively leading to a greater understanding of a systematic phenotype-genotype of the disorder (Hagberg *et al.* 2002).

Aetiology

It is estimated that RS affects 1:10,000 to 15,000 live female births across all ethnic groups. A genetic disorder, RS is caused by a severe gene mutation, a change in the DNA, or defects in the gene that encodes the Methyl-CpG-Binding Protein 2, or MECP2 impair gene transcription. The gene contains instructions to make a particular protein (MECP2) that is vital for brain development and the abnormality prevents nerve cells in the brain from working properly. However, evidence suggests less than 1 per cent of cases recorded are inherited, rather, most cases appear spontaneously, suggesting the gene mutation occurs randomly. Conversely too, some 80 per cent or more children fulfilling clinical criteria for RS may have MECP2 mutations, but such mutations may also be seen in children who do *not* have RS (Hagberg *et al.* 2002).

RS is often misdiagnosed as autism, cerebral palsy (CP) or non-specific developmental delay caused by a defective regulatory MECP2 gene found on the X chromosome. RS shows X-linked dominant inheritance and complete penetrance, or frequency of hereditary characteristics, but is notable for some variability in severity of clinical manifestations in the female, with two X chromosomes. Males have an X and a Y chromosome and common thinking until recently has construed that if there are flaws or defects in the X chromosome it is very likely that the male foetus would spontaneously abort. This view has been modified though to include boys who may survive with it, but be more severely affected than girls.

It is worth noting that since the initial criteria were established, remarkable progress has been made in the understanding of the clinical, neurobiological and molecular genetic characteristic of RS as a neurodevelopmental disorder. The prognosis though remains poor, there is no cure and the symptoms can be very difficult to manage. Mobility problems increase as the child moves into adolescence and feeding may also be a problem. Twenty-four-hour care will be needed for girls with RS, and throughout their lifespan. Their lifespan is shortened but many live into early and middle adulthood. Most boys with RS will have a very shortened lifespan.

Profile of features

RS is a degenerative disorder, characterized by normal development early on in life, followed by an arrest in development and subsequent regression in language and motor skills. Early onset of symptoms indicates presence of an autism disorder; and although investigations into other milder mutations in MECP2 gene predispose to autism, there are indications that mutation produces clinical features incompatible with RS. The science community, however, frequently locate RS on the autism spectrum. Diagnosis is tentative until the age of around 3–5 years. Criteria established from early research have over time been revised to clarify ambiguities in language.

Atypical development associated with classic RS

- Normal pre-natal and perinatal period: normal psychomotor development through first six months, and often 12–18 months of life.
- Normal head circumference at birth – deceleration of head growth (by inference, also brain growth) between six months and four years.
- Early behavioural, social and psychomotor regression (loss of achieved skills) development of communication dysfunction and signs of dementia.
- Loss of purposeful hand movements through ages 1–4 years, fine motor skills regress.
- Stereotypical repetitive hand motions, hand wringing as if hand washing.
- Intellectual development and resultant learning disabilities similar to those presented in autism disorders.
- May present with seizures.

Four stages of the disease are generally described but symptoms may overlap between each stage. They are:

- **Stage one – early signs and slow development** – age 6–18 months
  - a general slowness in development;
  - floppiness;
  - difficulty feeding;
  - less interest in social contact and eye contact;
  - not very interested in toys;
  - walking awkwardly and poor coordination of trunk and limbs.

- **Stage two – regression – rapid destructive stage** – age 1–4 years
  - repetitive and uncontrollable hand movements;
  - periods of distress, irritability and sometimes screaming for no obvious reason;
  - social withdrawal and loss of interest in people (may be considered as showing autistic behaviour);
  - unsteadiness of the body and awkward walking.

- **Stage three – plateau – can last for years** – age 2–10 years
  - floppiness of the limbs and difficulty moving around;
  - not being able to use hands to hold, carry or manipulate objects;
  - teeth grinding and abnormal tongue movements;
  - low and slow weight gain;
  - irregular breathing patterns, heart rhythm abnormalities;
  - 70 per cent of infants will develop epilepsy.

- **Stage four – deterioration in movement** – can last for years or decades
  - spine bending to the left or right side – scoliosis;
  - spasticity – abnormal stiffness in legs;
  - losing the ability to walk.

Making a diagnosis

- Clinical assessment and evaluation.

- Necessary diagnostic criteria for RS include:
  - female sex;
  - normal pre-natal and perinatal period through first six months;
  - normal head circumference at birth;
  - deceleration of head growth between age five months and four years;
  - loss of purposeful hand skills, communication dysfunction and social withdrawal age 6–30 months;
  - development of seriously impaired expressive and receptive language and severe psychomotor retardation;
  - hand wringing, squeezing, clapping/tapping, hand rubbing;
  - appearance of gait apraxia, disorder of movement between ages 1–4 years.
- The presence of clinical features are a good indication for genetic testing.
- EEG test that measures electrical activity in the brain. May be useful in making a diagnosis.

Supportive criteria

1 Breathing dysfunction
   - periodic apnoea during wakefulness;
   - intermittent hyperventilation;
   - breath-holding spells;
   - forced expulsion of air or saliva.
2 Electroencephalogram abnormalities.
3 Seizures.
4 Spasticity, often when associated with development of muscle wasting and dystonia or muscle contractions, twisting and abnormal postures.
5 Peripheral vasomotor disturbances.
6 Scoliosis.
7 Growth retardation.
8 Hypotrophy, progressive degeneration of an organ or tissue by loss of cells.
                                                         (Hagberg *et al.* 2002)

References are given at the end of this chapter to support further enquiry via a web search and research helpline.

Appropriate support or intervention

- Social and psychological support for the parent and family.
- A blood test can identify genetic abnormality that underlies the cause.
- Genetic counselling of female family members (see Chapter 2) *and* genetic counselling of families with a newly diagnosed RS child.
- Management with the following aids or treatments:
  - anti-epileptic medication to control seizures;
  - physiotherapy, use of back brace, possible surgery to prevent scoliosis;
  - OT to develop life skills such as dressing or feeding;
  - feeding tube and other feeding aids;
  - an ankle/foot leg brace;
  - hand splint to control hand movements where severe;
  - technology aids to support communication.

For an account of case studies on individuals with RS, and a review of the literature I recommend the following reference:

Ravn, K., G. Roende, M. Duno, K. Fuglsang, K. L. Eiklid, Z. Tumer, J. B. Nielsej and O. H. Skjeldal (2011). 'Two new Rett syndrome families and review of the literature: expanding the knowledge of MECP2 frameshift mutations.' *Orphanet Journal of Rare Diseases*, 6 (58). Downloaded from www.ojrd.com/content/6/1/58 (accessed 30 April 2013).

Further information is available from the NHS website www.nhs.uk/Conditions/Rett-syndrome (accessed 20 July 2013).

For a definitive list of criteria, exclusionary criteria and the variant delineation model of RS, see Hagberg, B., F. Hanefeld, A. Percy and O. Skjeldal (2002). 'An update on clinically applicable diagnostic criteria in Rett Syndrome'. Comments to Rett Syndrome Clinical Criteria Consensus Panel Satellite to European Paediatric Neurology Society Meeting. Baden Baden, Germany, 11 September 2001. *European Journal of Paediatric Neurology*, 6 (0611), 1–5.

Autism Spectrum Disorder (ASD)

Brief history

Autism spectrum disorder (ASD) is really an umbrella term that refers to a range or spectrum of conditions that share common characteristics. This includes HFA or AS, the description of which follows in this chapter. The incidence of children and young people with autism in the UK has been steadily increasing over the past three decades, and once thought to be low incidence, or relatively uncommon, it is no longer regarded as a rare disease (Frith and Hill 2003). Recent prevalence studies estimate that approximately 1 per cent of the UK population are affected (Baron-Cohen *et al.* 2009).

First recognized by Leo Kanner (1943), we know far more now following more than 50 years of enquiry, and yet the nature, origin and even the definition are still points of much discussion. Causality is still largely unknown but as research is expanding, so is our knowledge and understanding of the condition. Historically autism was hypothesized as being due to emotional dysfunction, poor attachment to the mother and even abnormal child-rearing practices were considered as attributing factors. The 'refrigerator mother' label, for mothers of children diagnosed with a spectrum disorder, was coined initially by Kanner who posited that autism was due not only to inherited genetic traits, but also a lack of warmth toward the infant among the mothers (and fathers).

Bettelheim (1967) pursued this theory and while consistently emphasizing nurture over nature, also further laid blame on absent or weak fathers. He saw autistic theories of behaviour as stemming from the emotional frigidity of the mother, a view that endured in the UK and elsewhere until the end of the 1970s. Thankfully that view has largely been eradicated and research has shown in more recent years that it is a neurodevelopmental, brain-based, genetic disorder. Research into autism has undergone a period of consolidation and guided by three major cognitive theories: *theory of mind* (ToM), *language and coherence* and *executive dysfunction*. Each of these I describe below. Although no two children with ASD are the same, they all face challenges when interacting and communicating with others.

Aetiology

Although the exact causes of ASD are still very much the concern of neuroscientific, genetic and neurobiological fields of study, we know there is no one cause. Research has offered explanations that implicate gene changes, or mutations; a combination of autism 'at-risk' genes and environmental factors; early brain development; brain growth patterns (Stanley-Cary *et al.* 2011); and different parts of the brain not communicating with each other in a typical, or regular, way.

The synaptic 'pruning' action in the developing brain, described in Chapter 2, may be a significant period in autism where lack of 'pruning' in the child's brain may, in some way, offer a link to causal explanations. A strong genetic basis to ASD has been established, although the interaction of several genes may be involved and researchers continue to investigate several compromised genes. High-risk factors would appear to be: advanced parental age at time of conception, maternal illness during pregnancy, birth difficulties and particularly periods of oxygen deprivation during the birth. I stress though that these factors, by themselves, are insufficient to cause autism, rather in combination with genetic risk factors, they may modestly increase the risk.

Some families may have multiple children diagnosed, and a milder phenotype has been observed in sibling relatives of individuals with ASD. Frequently one parent, usually the father (Bolte *et al.* 2007) may also present similar personality traits although he may never have been formally diagnosed.

Key points

- A neurodevelopmental disorder.
- Highly heritable-genetic links.
- Preponderance of males 5:1.
- Usually has an onset before the age of 30 months.
- Absence of/or inadequate development of language.
- Obsessive responses to the environment.
- Majority are intellectually impaired.
- No biological markers for diagnosis.
- Pervasive, neurological, intractable so no cure, *but autism can be managed.*

Profile of features: a pattern of characteristics

A child with an autistic disorder will very likely present with many of these early warning signs or features in the domains of social, communication, behaviour and sensory development. Be aware also that symptoms of other, co-morbid conditions, such as ADHD, dyspraxia, Tics or Tourette's, an involuntary movement or repetitive twitching of muscles or involuntary vocalizing, sometimes also presenting in ADHD, or even epilepsy, may also be present.

Social

- Child doesn't consistently respond to his/her name.
- Doesn't smile at parent/caregivers.
- Doesn't use gestures spontaneously, e.g. wave bye-bye, copy others waving.

- Lack of joint attention is one of the earliest signs of autism.
- Impairments in gaze following. This 'joint-attention' behaviour rapidly develops from 6–12 months of age in normal or typically developing children. In the child with an ASD this behaviour doesn't happen.
- Doesn't enjoy or engage in infant action games, e.g. peek-a-boo, pat-a-cake, etc.
- Doesn't show an interest in other children, tends to be a loner, not necessarily interested in friendships or group membership.
- Social interaction difficulties, inability to empathize, understand the feelings or emotions of others.

Communication

- Doesn't use gestures such as raising arms to be picked up, or extend arm to show s/he wants to reach something.
- Communication difficulties, unable to make sense of both verbal and non-verbal language communication, fails to take cues from body language or facial expressions or gestures.
- Doesn't use eye contact to get attention or communicate.
- When being read to doesn't point at pictures and look at the reader.
- Thought and imagination limitations in early years, thought, imagination and play are impaired, may become fixated with one toy, likely to be a spinning or shiny toy.
- Doesn't understand simple one-step instructions.
- Speech significantly delayed, when developed can be repetitive or echolalia, repeating the last word or sound heard.

Behaviour

- Intense and repetitive actions and/or obsessive interests that will become compulsive.
- Focuses narrowly on objects and activities such as turning the wheels of a toy car or lining up objects.
- Easily upset by change of routine or move from familiar surroundings, sets routines for things that become a dominant procedure pattern for daily living.
- Repeats body movements or can show unusual body movements such as walking on toes, hand flapping or back arching.

Sensory

- Sensory perceptions disordered and sensory integration of everyday sights, sounds, tastes, feelings or tastes may be painful, uncomfortable, disturbing or create high state of anxiety; sensitivity to sensory information.
- Highly sensitive, hyper-acute hearing can be upset by heightened sensory experiences such as loud noise, background humming noise or repetitive sounds.
- Oversensitive to certain fabrics against the skin, e.g. labels near the collar, or fabric or fibres that 'feel itchy' or uncomfortable.
- Feeding and dietary problems; texture and taste of certain foods can be problematic.

- Seeks sensory stimulation, e.g. deep pressure, vibrating objects such as a washing machine or watching light flicker.

Atypical behaviour, cognitive and psychological functioning

- Self-stimulatory behaviour, or 'stimming', such as flapping hands, rocking, spinning; for many children 'stimming' helps to manage anxiety or fear, anger or panic.
- 'Insistence on sameness', and resistance to change. Inflexible. These traits are the cause of severe behaviour problems, stress and anxiety in the child.
- A lack of social or emotional reciprocity (APA 1994).
- Meltdown or out of control characteristics: this loss of behavioural control can be a violent response to a place, situation or event that is uncomfortable or frightening to the child. Unexpected changes can be a trigger; a change in routine or change from a recognized sequence of events. A meltdown can be loud, frightening, risky or endanger the child's safety, frustrating and totally exhausting for both the child and those trying to pacify the child.
- Repeating words or phrases, echolalia, imitating last sounds or words heard, over and over.

Effective responses, what to do, or not do, to deal with ASD behaviours

- Always make the immediate environment for the child a safe environment.
- A parent log should be encouraged; to help identify 'triggers' in the child's environment or spot the pattern of events that lead to extreme behaviours or meltdown.
- Help the parent to recognize the sort of situations that are likely to increase the chances of a meltdown occurring; once identified either avoid such situations or encourage the parent to prepare the child well in advance.
- Prepare strategies to set up an escape route or escape plan that will allow the child to be removed from any situation that is going to cause a potential problem.
- Work with the family to help them cope with adverse autistic behaviours.
- The use of weighted blankets, vests or other weighted items is recommended: weighted items are items such as vests, blankets, cushions or toys that are filled with weights such as sand, rice or wheat and used to provide sustained, deep pressure which is believed to be calming. Weighted blankets have been found to help manage restlessness in children with sensory integration dysfunction that is a characteristic of both ASD and ADHD. Weighted items have been found effective as they provide the calming, deep pressure input that those with ASD frequently respond to.
- Use clear precise language. Language may be interpreted literally so instructions need to be clear and precise. Avoid idioms, nuances, inference, puns, metaphors and sarcasm. These cannot be understood. The child with AS will need to have instructions clearly expressed, repeated and sequential instructions kept to a minimum.
- Emotional language may be difficult to decode, and the child may not have the emotional literacy to describe feelings or moods. Emotional literacy is discussed in more detail in later chapters (see Chapters 6 and 9).

- Routine-based interventions to promote the social reciprocity of young children with autism, undertaken in the child's natural environments. Parent training can be used during everyday routines and activities, to help parents and other caregivers establish long chains of back-and-forth interactions with young children with autism.

Prominent theories and research

ToM is our capacity to understand mental states, or the way we imagine other people's feelings or thoughts. It is important because 'the ability to make inferences about what other people believe to be the case in a given situation allows one to predict what they will do' (Baron-Cohen *et al.* 1985: 39). This is an essential capacity if we are to develop empathy, and appreciate the feelings, opinions, thoughts and even actions of others. One test used in psychological research to investigate ToM in children is the 'Sally-Anne test' (see Appendix 1), a simple activity that has, over the years, presented support for autistic children lacking a ToM. It is also now posited that a lack of it may explain some of the social and communication difficulties experienced by individuals with autism (Tager-Flusberg 2007).

Central coherence theory is the weak central coherence theory of autism (Frith 1989) that describes the human being's inability to gain meaning out of a mass of information or details. A person with a strong central coherence would view the overall incoming information and from it deduce meaning (Rippon *et al.* 2007). An individual with a weak central coherence would only see the massive input of confusing information and be unable to make any sense of it. In ASD the brain receives huge amounts of information, but a defective filtering system allows an overload to occur, and thus lead to a meltdown situation. The meltdown is a common characteristic of autism and, unlike a temper tantrum, where a child may use the social situation to their benefit, in a meltdown the child does not look, or care, about the reactions of others to this behaviour. The meltdown is a total loss of control that completely overwhelms the child.

Executive function impediment in ASD is an associated executive dysfunction theory. It makes the connection between deficits in autism in the domains of mental processing that help to connect past experience to present actions (Happé *et al.* 2006). This is evidenced in, for example, planning, organizing, attending, focusing and shifting attention, and the development of understanding. Frith (1989) considered that other theories of ASD might account for core deficits in cognitive functioning, but that they failed to take account of 'savant' traits that often present. Savant traits are exceptional skills in memory, music, art and/or mathematics that interestingly are not exhibited in many non-autistic or neurotypical (NT) individuals. The prevalence of savant traits in the NT population is usually given as less than 1 per cent but the prevalence of 'savant' talents in the autistic population is approximately 10 per cent.

Extreme male brain theory – systematizing /empathizing – Simon Baron-Cohen (2002) proposed two brain types, an empathic female brain that, on average, more women would present with, and a systematizing male brain that, on average, more men would have. People with autism, Baron-Cohen suggests, have trouble reading not just thoughts, but also feelings and lack a strong 'empathetic' sense. The male brain though is defined psychometrically as having 'systemizing' strengths. In this framework, people with autism could be seen to possess an extreme male brain (Baron-Cohen 2002). There is increasing psychological evidence for this theory and this could also, possibly, account for the preponderance of males with autism. Linked to this is what takes place during the development of the foetus, where possibly the development of an extreme male could be the result of exposure to high levels of fetal testosterone. This provides another interesting theory and research at Cambridge University in the UK is exploring this pathway (Auyeung *et al.* 2009).

Genetic predisposition for autism continues to be investigated with a strong emphasis on a combination of genetic and environmental factors, but also a strong unambiguous genetic component that may explain the 'at-risk' connection. It may also be that no one primary gene is an associated causal factor, rather, it is more likely to be a number of different genetic variants that increase the risk (Schaefer and Lutz 2006).

Gastro-intestinal problems in autism and gut problems have been implicated as a causal factor in ASD, with links made to the yeast form *Candida Albicans* and investigative links between symptoms, believed to be due to faecal bacteria, with a higher incidence also of the *Clostridium Histolyticum* bacteria group found in individuals with autism, than was found in healthy typical children (Parracho *et al.* 2005). Gastrointestinal abnormalities are also linked to theories that include inflammation in the upper and lower intestinal tracts. Studies with exclusionary diets, eliminating intakes of gluten and casein have also been investigated, and suggest digestive problems associated with derivative gluten and casein peptides are a causal factor, associated directly with an immune response in children with ASD. I discuss dietary treatments further in Chapter 8.

Different brain development

- In children with autism aberrant growth rates in areas of the brain implicated in the social impairment, communication deficits and repetitive behaviours have been found; these being characteristic features of autism.
- Slower growth of the brain in ASD extends into adolescence (Courchesne *et al.* 2001).
- The brain of a child with ASD appears to have more cells and inefficient connections between the cells (e.g. a lack of pruning?).

Making a diagnosis

During the first-year monitoring recommended under the HCP, a child's social development is of particular significance when looking for early signs of an ASD. Particular behaviours to look for are lack of smiling, eye contact, babbling and developing pre-language sounds. Signs are usually seen in the first two years. Some children will display many of the warning signs, others may only present with a few, but any baby showing developmental anomalies, or *any* abnormalities, should be referred early to a specialist team.

There are no available medical tests for autism. An accurate diagnosis must therefore be based on observations of the child's communication, behaviour and developmental levels. However, since many of the behaviours associated with autism are shared by other disorders, an experienced clinician may perform various tests to rule out, or identify, other possible causes of the symptoms being exhibited. A pediatrician or child and adolescent psychiatrist will make the final diagnosis. Examples of screening instruments are described below, but it is stressed here that a comprehensive developmental history from the family, HV and any other health or social care professional involved with the child is also crucial.

Autism Diagnostic Observation Schedule (ADOS) (Lord *et al.* 2001) is an instrument for diagnosing and assessing autism through a series of semi-structured tasks that demand social interaction between the tester and the test taker. The tester observes and classifies segments of a child's behaviour and assigns them to categories that are subsequently combined to produce quantitative scores for analysis. It allows for a standardized assessment of autistic symptoms and is suitable for use with children from 12 months of age. The age range for which it is said to be appropriate is from toddler, or child with no speech through to adults who are verbally fluent.

Autism Diagnostic Interview, Revised ADI-R (Rutter *et al.* 2003) is an instrument that is not only for diagnosis and planning treatment in the child with autism, but also distinguishes autism from other developmental disorders. It is a standardized interview schedule, of 93 questions, spanning the domains of language and communication, reciprocal social interactions, and restricted, repetitive and stereotyped behaviour and interests. The ADI-R test is suitable for use with children from around the age of two years and up to adult.

Social Responsiveness Scale (SRS) (Constantino and Gruber 2005) is a 65-item rating scale and a quantitative measure of autistic traits in children aged from two and a half years up to adults. It measures the severity of autism spectrum symptoms as they occur in natural social settings. It is a widely used parent–teacher report measure of autistic traits for use in the general population, and in clinical and educational settings. It generates an index of deficiency in social reciprocity, rather than providing a characterization of symptoms present or a given disorder. It also gives a clear indication of a child's social impairments, social awareness, social information processing capacity for reciprocal social communication, social anxiety/avoidance, and autistic preoccupations and traits.

Childhood Autism Rating Scale (CARS2) (Schopler *et al.* 2010) is a structured interview and observation instrument used to assess children suspected of having an autism spectrum disorder. It helps to identify children with autism and distinguishes them from developmentally delayed children who are *not* autistic. Additionally, it distinguishes through a rating scale that derives an overall score, the degree or severity of the impact from mild to moderate or severe autism. It is deemed suitable for use with children from age two years and onwards.

Appropriate interventions

There is no known cure for autism but many programmes and strategies can be used to manage core symptoms or difficulties the child and families may experience. Major difficulties in social interaction are consistently identified as a central feature of autism interventions. Strategies to address social skills and social behaviour are therefore usually identified as the first area on which to focus. Below a sample of intervention techniques that have been found to be effective are described.

- **Naturalistic techniques:** typically employ behaviour methods to deliver therapy in everyday settings. Using naturally occurring antecedents and consequences – or ABC method – *antecedent*, *behaviour* and *consequences* – has shown to be successful with early years and pre-school children; it usually also involves using another technique as well.

- **Social Stories™** (www.thegraycenter.org/social-stories) accurately describe a situation, skill or relevant social cues that you want the child to learn. They do not aim to modify behaviour, rather they should aim to improve understanding of social events and social situations (www.thegraycenter.org).
- **Parent training** trains parents to deliver the therapy services to the child.
- **Peer training or peer mediation** involves practitioners training age-matched peers to deliver direct intervention techniques to the child with ASD.
- **Social skills groups** involve two or more age-matched individuals with and/or without an ASD to receive instruction central to which are specific social skills or social competence and to work with the child with an ASD to improve his/her social interaction skills.
- **Visual training** involves the use of picture cues, social stories or visual 'scripts' to model desired social behaviour and/or undesirable behaviour. Typically an adult delivers interventions using visual techniques to the child with ASD. This builds on a strength/ability that many individuals with ASD have, being able to visualize something or think in pictures. Many children with ASD think in pictures and this strategy may show the child the ways they can develop greater social understanding about situations, protocols and social interaction 'norms'.
- **Video modelling** involves the presentation of video vignettes, or situations, to the child with an ASD using a television or computer monitor. Social stories can also be used as 'scripts' here and ideally this will model behaviour that focuses on where behavioural changes or modifications are needed.
- **Applied Behavioural Analysis (ABA)** is an approach that employs behavioural intervention to build positive behaviour, encourage communication and suppress unwanted behaviour such as aggression. A 'lack of social or emotional reciprocity' is listed as one of the 16 possible characteristics of autism in the *DSM-IV* (APA 1994) and this refers to the social give-and-take between individuals involved in an interaction. For example, you smile at your child and they smile back. You give affection and receive an affectionate response. For slightly older children it includes chatting back and forth. This back-and-forth social exchange between two people I described earlier (see Chapter 1) and is what Bronfenbrenner (1979) termed as a game of human 'ping-pong'.

    For the child with autism, social and emotional reciprocity needs to be acquired with something more than chance; reciprocity needs to be developed more purposefully by non-autistics and applied more generously *towards* autistics, and ABA is underpinned by this notion. ABA is believed to improve social, communication and skills of daily living, while also helping to reduce difficult behaviours. I return to the concept of reciprocity again in Chapter 9.

Applied treatments are numerous and the following are intended as a sample. Their inclusion here is not intended to endorse their efficacy, or recommend one above another but I add here that professionals should always have a clear understanding of what an intervention is claiming, what evidence there is to support the claim, who is making the claims and what is their interest (e.g. marketing a product or having a vested interest from which they will profit). I revisit and expand on this and the issue of parent vulnerability regarding intervention treatments in Chapter 8.

- **Treatment and Education of Autistic and related Communication handicapped Children (TEACCH)** is described as a combined type of therapy that aims to identify the child's strengths and skills, and to promote learning and development in children with ASD. It creates and builds a very structured learning environment, is intensive and helps children to understand how daily life works so they can become more independent. The programme is for individuals with autism of all ages from child through to adults.

- **Developmental Social Pragmatic Model (DSP)** is an approach to promote communication that employs everyday interactions between caregivers and the child with ASD. Its aim is to build on basic communication skills the child may have, it is derived from ABA and is based on developmental theory and research on interactions between typically developing children and their caregivers. In a DSP framework all communication efforts, verbal or non-verbal, are rewarded.

- **CBT, counselling, psychotherapy** are underpinned by the idea that how we think, feel and act affects each other. Reducing high anxiety, teaching coping strategies and dealing with relationship issues are just some areas that CBT can embrace and improve.

Many of the issues raised in the discussion of ASD can also be recognized in the child with AS, but there are also some subtle differences and these I will highlight below.

Further information can be found on the NAS website www.autism.org.uk and at www.nhs.uk/conditions/autistic-spectrum-disorder.

Further recommended reading

Baron-Cohen, S., Tager-Flsberg, H. and Cohen, D. (2000). *Understanding other Minds: Perspectives from Developmental Cognitive Neuroscience*. Oxford, Oxford University Press.
Frith, U. and Frith, C. (2003). 'Development and neurophysiology of mentalizing'. *Philosophical Transactions of the Royal Society B: Biological Sciences*, 358, 459–473.
Ruffman, T., Garnham, W. and Rideout, P. (2001). 'Social understanding in autism: eye gaze as a measure of core insights'. *Journal of Child Psychology and Psychiatry*, 42, 1083–1094.

Asperger Syndrome (AS)/High-Functioning Autism (HFA)

Brief historical perspective

AS is also known as HFA but will be referred to as AS in this analysis. To be clear though the two terms are referring to the same thing. On the spectrum of autism disorders over the past three decades, AS has moved from relative obscurity to high-profile status. Public awareness has been raised and AS has been given much media attention. Knowledge about the condition has also increased through advancements in scientific and medical research. The substantial increase in the prevalence of autism necessitates that practising physicians, health and community nurses become more familiar with the presentation of symptoms, and this undoubtedly will support improved early diagnoses rates and thus earlier application of interventions. In the longer-term, this can only improve the prognosis for affected children and their families.

A developmental disability, AS affects the way the child develops and understands the world around them. It is directly linked to the information conveyed by the senses and sensory processing. Information bombards the individual, too much at any one time for the individual to process, as an impaired filtering system fails to regulate input. It is said that the child with ASD lives in his or her own world, but the child with AS lives in this world, *differently*. The child often uses egocentric 'quirky' behaviours (e.g. spinning or repetitive habituated behaviour) to block out their emotions or in response to anxiety or pain.

The condition was first described by Han Asperger who, in 1944, provided a description of clinical features that were very similar to those present in autism described by Kanner in 1943, a year earlier. These shared features were difficulties with social interaction and communication and intense focus on idiosyncratic interest. However, there were also distinct differences between autism and AS. Delay in acquiring speech was not always present in what Asperger was describing, compared to Kanner's autism features. Speech difficulties were less common and a strong genetic feature was present, with other family members showing similar traits or features of AS and frequently this being the father. Children with AS usually have average or above average IQ. This is not the case in ASD. The child with HFA is often described as 'twice exceptional' as they may have an exceptional talent *and* AS.

AS was first recognized in the UK in 1981 through case study research by Lorna Wing (Wing 1981) and following the evaluation of Asperger's work. It first appeared in the *ICD* manual (see Chapter 3) in 1991 and the *DSM-IV* in 1994. However, it was removed as a separate disorder in the *DSM-5* (2013) for reasons given earlier (see Chapter 3). It is often referred to as HFA because of specialized areas of interest, where an enormous amount of information is obsessively acquired through the individual's special interest.

Children with AS will often speak in a monotonous or exaggerated tone and at great length about things. This means they are frequently referred to as 'boffin, nerd or geek'. They may sound far more adult than their chronological age, and although able to talk seemingly knowledgably, it will be on a restricted topic of their specific interest. In young children the obsession is often with animated versions of the Reverend W Awdry's character *Thomas the Tank Engine*. Indeed, in 2001 an NAS survey of parents of children with AS found:

- these children associate far more strongly with *Thomas the Tank Engine* than with other children's characters;
- the children maintained their association on average two years longer than typically developing children; and
- that almost one-third of the parents considred AS as an obsessive relationship with, for example, a comfort blanket or even a friend.

Explanations given as to 'why *Thomas*' include:

- calm and clear narration through each story;
- alerts the child overtly to any change in the plot;
- stories follow a typical pattern, and all problems are solved by the end of each story;
- the trains are the only things that move, the scenery stays in place;

- slow, often exaggerated facial expressions can teach children to recognize emotions; and
- *Thomas* can encourage 'pretend play'.

If you Google 'Autism and Thomas the Tank Engine' in 0.28 seconds 617,000 results are thrown up. As such *Thomas* can be a useful point of entry both for the initial professional/child interaction, and to the world of communication and learning.

Aetiology

A lifelong disability, AS affects how a person makes sense of the world, processes information and relates to other people. There is no cure but it can change over time with continued training, support and maturation. It may vary in degrees of severity across a spectrum, but behavioural approach is the mainstay of therapy to address the core symptoms. No specific brain pathology has been described and where subtle brain differences have been found, they are not restricted to one particular brain region (Bauman and Kemper 2005). Although it remains unclear whether autism is a distinctly separate disorder to AS, it has been suggested, and shown, that motor deficits, and particularly cerebellar activity, may be different. In addition, potentially, differential neurobiological substrates may underpin the two complex disorders (Stanley-Cary *et al.* 2011).

There may be some slight variance, but children with AS tend to present with similar symptoms. There is a strong gender bias with more prevalence among boys. Girls can also have the condition, although statistically less often than boys. Asperger himself thought it could not be recognized in infancy, usually not before the third year of life or later, but with developments in neuroscientific knowledge and from extant research, we can now identify traits that sound alarm bells when developmentally something untoward begins to become apparent before the age of 30 months. As with other disorders described (e.g. dyspraxia), it is mostly a hidden disability, as at first meeting you can't immediately tell that someone has the condition. Spend any time with the child or adult with AS, however, and it soon becomes apparent that something is 'not quite right'.

Profile of features and characteristics

- Difficulties with social functioning, particularly social communication, social interaction and social imagination.
- Sensory issues, oversensitive to noise, bright lights, unpleasant smells, some fabrics.
- Obsessive interests with a focus on one subject to the exclusion of all others.
- A rigid resistance to change in routine, 'insistence on sameness' (Ollington *et al.* 2012); reaction to sudden change can lead to an emotional and physiological meltdown.
- Social isolation, struggles with friendship relationships, lack of empathy, failing to take social cues, understand social protocols or understand about didactic relationships.
- Naïve and gullible so also vulnerable.
- Habituation; a need for order in their everyday life.
- Difficulties in expressing themselves emotionally and socially.
- Physically awkward, gross motor skills performed clumsily.

Atypical behaviours

- Idiosyncratic 'quirky' behaviours that set them apart from peers because they are seen as 'odd'.
- Inflexibility; unusually accurate memory for details.
- Sleeping or eating problems.
- Oversensitivity to sensory information, sight, sounds, smells, tastes and touch.
- Trouble comprehending things – very literal.
- Inappropriate body language or facial expression.
- Tendency to rock or fidget.
- Dwells on minutiae – fixations on one subject or thing.
- May have tics, involuntary rapid or sudden movement or sound, repeated over and over again; blinking, coughing or sniffing repeatedly and excessively, or spinning.

Strengths

- May be highly intelligent *but not always*.
- SL develop early, often before walking.
- May learn to read without specific instruction, but just seem to acquire reading, or decoding skills sometimes even before instruction has begun: stores away long words to use in conversation although not often understanding what they mean.
- Honest: people with AS *cannot* lie, they do not know how.
- Highly accurate episodic and long-term memory often recalling minute detail associated with an event or experience, e.g. the colour of the shoes/coat/shirt someone wore at a first meeting.

Weaknesses

- Inflexible, must stick to known routines.
- Social skills, interaction skills, may fail to initiate or sustain social relationships this *may cause them anxiety but not always*.
- Frequently lives in a heightened state of anxiety.
- Thought processes often confined to a narrow, pedantic, literal but often a logical chain of reasoning.
- Appearing aloof or unfriendly with other children or some adults. Often leading to poor perceptions, or judgement, about them (e.g seen as unfriendly, unapproachable or arrogant individuals).

Prominent theories

- Genetic disorder strong hereditary links, multiple genes are implicated. NO genetic test available to identify marker genes. Heritability high genetics explains over 90 per cent of whether a child will develop AS (extrapolated estimate from twin studies; Freitag 2007).
- Several mutations found that may cause the disorder, some siblings do not carry it, females much more resistant to the effects of mutations, which may be one reason autism is much more prevalent in boys.

- Environmental factors, e.g. heavy metal toxicity, chemicals in the home environment.
- Viral infection during gestation, and exposure to teratogens as in FASDs.
- Gluten and casein allergic reactions, inflammation of the gut.

Important in the prominent theory debate concerns infant reactions to vaccinations, particularly the triple component vaccination for Mumps, Measles and Rubella (MMR). Andrew Wakefield published a paper citing manipulated false data to make claims that falsely attributed this as a causal explanation in 1998. This theory has been empirically dismissed and Wakefield was removed from the medical register after being found guilty of malpractice in 2010. However, new parents may still attach some credence to this causal hypothesis and, understandably, show concerns that the health professional will need to address from an informed stance.

Making a diagnosis

Making a diagnosis can be complicated and there is a lack of available standardized diagnostic instruments specifically for AS. There are screening tests, some of which are described in the ASD diagnostic tools above, but each instrument has different criteria and lacks specificity. Depending on which test it would not be impossible for the same child to be given several different diagnoses. Referral to paediatrician or child and adolescent psychiatrist is strongly advised. Using a diagnostic manual as described in Chapter 3, the child must show certain specific traits. For example from the *DSM-IV* two of the following traits or problems would need to be present:

- Marked impairment regarding non-verbal social cues, e.g. does not make eye contact/understand others' body language.
- Fails to make friends.
- Lack of appropriate social and emotional responses to others; or inability to spontaneously share enjoyment, interests and achievements with other people.

In addition, the child must show one of the following:

- An abnormal or intense interest in one subject.
- Strictly adhering to a set of self-inflicted own rules, routines and rituals.
- Repeating certain mannerisms like hand flapping, hair twisting or whole body movement.
- An obsession in the mechanical parts of objects.

Ideally a two-stage process should be involved, with the first stage being developmental screening as part of the universal progressive reviews as recommended in the HCP. Where autistic features become apparent in the developmental process and concerns are shared between parents and professionals, this should be followed with a referral for a comprehensive examination by a professional who has expertise in diagnosing children with AS or ASD. A multi-agency approach to manage symptoms may be required, such as occupational therapist, physiotherapist and/or speech therapist, and/or clinical psychologist.

Appropriate intervention

I would like to make the point here that if a child has any disorder on the autism spectrum, professionals should first and foremost always try to refer to the child as 'a child that has autism' as it is only one aspect of the overall character of the child. Professionals need to know and understand the label does *not* define the child as a person. The child may *have* autism, but is *not* first and foremost an autistic child. Defining a child by a characteristic or label may be setting up a low expectation.

Intervention should fundamentally be a planned, structured and coordinated programme that begins with parent training, but should also share some of the features below.

- A predictable and regular timetable.
- Be sequential and accumulative, each step building on the previous, highly structured activities, regularly reinforcing desired outcomes.
- Social skills training, therapy group sessions teaching rules and conventions of social interaction/turn taking and social cues.
- Behaviour therapy to work through inflexible traits; behavioural flexibility is what should underpin any planned programme of behaviour.
- CBT to manage high anxiety, obsessive interests and emotions better.
- Medication may be necessary if anxiety and depression are serious – perhaps in the adolescence period of development.
- Occupational therapy (OT) or physiotherapy where sensory integration problems are severely impeding social functioning (e.g. taking clothes off when in an inappropriate social situation) or poor motor coordination is evident.
- Specialist SLT where SPD affects communication or social interacting.

Additional reading

The following texts are recommended for further information:

Attwood, T. (2006). *The Complete Guide to Asperger Syndrome*. London, Jessica Kingsley Publishers.
Clements, J. (2005). *People with Autism Behaving Badly*. London, Jessica Kingsley Publishers.
Delfos, M.F. (2005). *A Strange World: Autism, Asperger's Syndrome and PDD-NOS*. London, Jessica Kingsley Publishers.
Roth, I. (2010). *The Autism Spectrum in the 21st Century: Exploring Psychology, Biology and Practice*. London, Jessica Kingsley Publishers.

Websites: Asperger Foundation www.aspergerfoundation.org.uk (accessed 29 July 2013).

Willams-Beuren Syndrome (WS/WBS)

Brief history

Williams Syndrome is also known as Williams-Beuren Syndrome but the condition here will be referred to here as Williams Syndrome (WS). WS is a rare neurodevelopmental genetic disorder that occurs because of a deletion, or missing piece, of genetic material. It was described independently as two seemingly unrelated disorders. First by a New Zealand cardiologist and colleagues (Williams *et al.* 1961) who in a seminal paper described four patients as having cardiac problems, mental or cognitive disabilities, shortness in stature, with specific 'elfin' facial features, wide-spaced eyes, a wide-set mouth, and presenting as gregarious and very friendly. A year later German physicians (Beuren *et al.* 1962) reported similar features to those described by Williams *et al.* in three patients but it wasn't until 1993 that the genetic connection to the disorder was confirmed (Morris *et al.* 1993). Study of this rare syndrome over the past 50 years has contributed broadly to the knowledge about the structure and function of extra cellular matrix, genomic structures and rearrangement involved in this condition, as well as beginning to describe genetic underpinnings of learning, language and behaviour. Research is also underpinning the development of interventions that can be successfully implemented.

Aetiology

WS is a rare genetic disorder. It occurs because of a deletion, or missing piece, of genetic material on chromosome 7 and is due to a random error when either the sperm or the egg was forming. The absent material includes the gene that controls the production of elastin, a protein that provides elasticity and suppleness to various structures in the body, including skin and blood vessel walls. Those children with much longer deletions typically have a more severe phenotype; individuals with shorter deletions will have a less severe subset of signs and symptoms.

WS is inherited in an autosomal dominant way, a pattern of inheritance in which an affected individual has one copy of a mutant gene on a pair of autosomal chromosomes. Thus the individual with such a disease as WS would have a 50:50 chance of passing the mutant gene, and therefore WS, onto each of their children, although most people with WS do not reproduce. The risk to parents of having another child with WS is no higher than the original risk, and the risk of siblings parenting a child with WS is also not increased. The condition occurs randomly and as a result of new genetic change that occurs at the time of conception. It must be stressed that the syndrome is not linked to anything the parents did, or did not do, during the pregnancy. Genetic counselling can be reassuring in the event of another planned child or for the siblings when they are wishing to have a child themselves.

It has an estimated prevalence range given approximately as from one in 7,500, one in 10,000 and even one in 20,000 births, depending on the country reporting and how current the information is. As more is learned about this disorder then the more cases will be recognized. It affects boys and girls alike, and is found across all races and in all countries. It is a specific disorder with specific traits or features. It is intractable and with no cure; produces distinctive physical features; can be detected through blood and gene pathology; and may present many physical, developmental, intellectual and social problems for the individual and his/her family that will require multi-agency services from post-natal through to the longer term. Independent living is not a realistic outcome.

Profile of features

WS has a characteristic constellation of physical, physiological and neurodevelopmental features. As with all developmental disorders, however, the extent of medical and developmental problems is highly variable. In infancy they may present early in the neonate as an irritable baby with feeding and digestion problems and that does not thrive well.

Physical features

- Distinctive facial 'elfin' features, iris 'star' bright eyes, small chin, generous lips, upturned nose/flat nose bridge.
- Weight and growth problems; possible low birth weight and slow weight gain.
- Feeding and swallowing difficulties.
- Unusual dental and palate shapes, small teeth, widely spaced and misaligned bite.
- Hyperacusis – hypersensitive hearing.

Physiological anomalies

- Predisposition to cardiovascular defects, narrowed aorta-aortic stenosis, narrowed pulmonary artery-pulmonary stenosis; valve abnormalities.
- Endocrine abnormalities that include hypercalcemia or high levels of calcium in the blood.
- Thyroid abnormalities; diabetes mellitus.
- Poor infant feeders; colic and problems chewing and swallowing.
- Gastroesophageal reflux; diverticular disease and often childhood inguinal hernia.

Neurodevelopmental cognitive and perceptual features

- Difficulty with visua-spatial construction.
- Cognitive limitations, low ability but IQ range from 40 to 100 found, mean IQ approximately 55; characteristic pattern of cognitive strengths and weaknesses that gives a WS cognitive profile.
- Socially exuberant, friendly, talk happily to strangers.
- Mastery of expressive language usually far earlier than typically developing peers.
- Total lack of social inhibition, gregarious, friendly, uninhibited and vulnerable.
- Delayed motor skill development; coordination problems.

Personality, social, emotional and behavioural well-being

- Interacts well with adults and peers but lacks social inhibition or awareness of social protocols or situations.
- Enjoyment of music is universal–paradoxical as they are sensitive to certain noises, e.g. load aircraft or traffic, thunderstorms, fireworks.
- Impressive social and verbal skills.
- Challenged by visua-spatial-perceptual activities such as jigsaw puzzles or construction tasks.

Strengths

- Highly social and empathetic.
- Good social and interpersonal skills.
- Auditory rote memory.
- Good facial recognition.

Weaknesses

- Delayed toilet training.
- Vomiting, constipation and/or diarrhoea.
- Recurrent bladder and urinary tract infections.
- Impulsive and short attention span (ADHD).
- Prone to anxieties and phobias; obsessive and/or compulsive behaviours and interests.
- Musculoskeletal problems; lax joints, scoliosis.

Making a diagnosis

Clinical diagnosis is possible using criteria if the health professional is an astute observer; laboratory pathology testing is rapid, accurate and conclusive.

- Clinical diagnosis based on diagnostic testing the Fluoriscent in situ hybridization (FISH) test.
- Blood test can determine if levels of calcium in the blood are high – hypercalcemia.
- MRI brain scanning studies have delineated neurologic underpinnings distinct to WS (Morris 2010). Not a readily available option in the UK yet.

Appropriate intervention, treatment and/or management

Treatment will involve a range of multi-agency care and support. There is no cure and the medical physician or paediatrician is the primary or key figure in advocated and implementation of any intervention programme. Depending on symptoms presented treatment can include:

- surgery to correct physiological defects in cardiac structure/gut/renal structures;
- regular medical monitoring;
- dental or orthodontic treatment;
- physical therapy from physiotherapist/OT;
- social training;
- speech therapy;
- pharmacotherapy;
- family genetic counselling;
- integrated services to support the family with a range of multi-agencies.

Additional information can be obtained from:

- The Williams Syndrome Foundation UK www.williams-syndrome.org.uk (accessed 20 July 2013).
- www.cafamily.org.uk/medical-information/conditions/w/williams-syndrome (accessed 20 July 2013).
- Semel, E. and Rosner, S. R. (2011). *Understanding Williams Syndrome: Behavioural Patterns and Interventions.* London, Routledge, Taylor & Francis Library.

Activity 5.1: SAQs

As the last two chapters have shown, many disorders described share some common features of which 16 are listed below. This exercise will summarize for you some features, or characteristics above, that *could*, but *may not*, be present in each of the conditions given in the list (a) to (g).

e.g. ADHD (1) (4) (5) (7) (8) (9) (10) (11) (12)

Features or characteristics

1   Easily distracted and forgetful.
2   Will not make eye contact when spoken to.
3   Hand flapping, spinning or rocking.
4   Language development irregular.
5   Unable to focus on any one thing.
6   Is most commonly found in girls.
7   Is most commonly found in boys (but not exclusively).
8   Problems achieving developmental milestones.
9   Difficulty understanding spatial concepts.
10 Poorly coordinated.
11 Inability to recognize potential danger.
12 Late mastering puzzles that require fine motor coordination.
13 Speaks fluently in a grown up way.
14 Heightened sensitivity to sounds and noises.
15 Fixates on certain topics.
16 Is degenerative.

Disorders

a   ASD/AS;
b   dyspraxia;
c   dyslexia;
d   ADHD;
e   RS;
f   FASD;
g   WBS.

Summary

* Although the disorders are described as 'low incidence' or 'low frequency' and may appear less frequently than disorders described in the previous chapter, advances in knowledge mean that more cases are being identified. This is *not* the same as an increase, or endemic rise, in the prevalence of a condition.

- The trajectory for each condition, theoretical causality and appropriate intervention or treatment to manage behaviour that is manifest, are specific to each disorder, but overlapping features can be observed as Activity 5.1 demonstrates.
- Professionals need to take into account that no two children with the same disorder will necessarily present with the same difficulties; but within the difficulties a pattern or profile of core features can be present.
- Specific complexities need to be investigated with each individual case. Always consider the similarities as well as the differences when making a diagnosis.
- A positive functioning outcome can be achieved, with a consistent holistic approach, consultation with parents and all professionals, and that is essentially centred on, and around, the child.

Note

1 For research and access to medical and international resources, use the medical spelling 'fetal'.

Part 3

Application to practice

Working in partnership, meeting all needs

Overview

In earlier chapters, the case for a multi-disciplinary approach to study human development was made. It was stressed that the child be in a pivotal role for any planned intervention or treatment; the issue of safeguarding was, and continues to be, raised throughout, so too was the point made concerning how we access the views of the child (Chapter 1), and take their views, wishes and feelings into account in any decision concerning him or her. Legislation and government guidance has been outlined, and aligned to the protection, vulnerability and rights of children, young people and families. Professional codes of ethics were discussed. Normal or typical developmental patterns were described (Chapter 2), and developmental surveillance points, screening and diagnostic assessment procedures and their significance were delineated (Chapter 3), particularly when considering how to identify and meet the specific needs of children with the described disorders and conditions (Chapters 4 and 5).

The chapters in Part 3 represent a shift in emphasis. Here the focus is on the application to practice, working in partnerships to meet the needs of a child or family affected by a developmental disorder, within health, education and social policy. It looks to identify the constraints and demands embedded within systems described in the social modelling framework presented in Chapter 1. First, in the chapter that follows (Chapter 6) psychological and socialization issues, the secondary impact and frequent consequence of a congenital developmental disorder are discussed, and linked to developmental theories discussed earlier (see Chapter 2). Patterns of vulnerability and manifest secondary effects of a developmental disorder are explored in the context of those 'at risk' of poor psychosocial functioning and mental health problems. The distinction is made between a mental problem and a mental disorder; the manifest secondary issues that may arise. Examples of intervention treatment and support agencies that are available for young people are described, and the role of the CAMHS is also considered. Safeguarding children and young people with disabilities or compromised maturation because of a developmental condition is discussed, and professional responsibilities for child protection for those with additional needs and their families are outlined. This chapter closes with a summing up of the skills and knowledge necessary for HVs, nurses and other agents involved at the frontline of service delivery, if they are to identify and address, through intervention, potential psychosocial problems in children and young people.

Chapter 7 looks at meeting needs from the perspective of the child or young person. The structure of the environment model introduced in Chapter 1 (Bronfenbrenner 1979) is the framework for analysis. Ever-changing variables within the systems are the focus of enquiry framed here and some of the impacting factors affecting a national framework that act to impede early diagnosis or early intervention are identified. Where the child has an adverse developmental trajectory, meeting additional support needs can mean professionals are constantly faced with opposing tensions. Some such tensions and conflicts of interest inherent within systems in England are identified here. If changes to be implemented are to be truly 'child friendly', inclusive and meet all legal demands, it follows that the views, voices and experiences of *all* children and young people with learning difficulties and/or disabilities must be considered. The issue of accessing the child's voice is explored here and evidence presented to show what children and young people are saying. Strategies that have a child and young person focus to support communication, listening *and* hearing are explored. Under legislative change in England, the young person is 'the client' and the family, the consumers, purchase support services through personal budget or direct payment of SEN funding. The complex issue of financing universal health, care and support is then introduced, and international trends in funding formulas and allocation of resources are explored.

In Chapter 8, the parent's perspective is the focus. I begin by presenting one LA's response to providing a cost-effective, multi-professional model of collaborative working with the family. The case study of good practice is presented in the SA. I then look at parent vulnerability, where their children have an adverse developmental trajectory, and the role of the professional as an advisor on 'fads' or 'miracle cures'. A sample of treatments for specific learning difficulties (e.g. dyslexia, ADHD, autism) once popularized and considered radical, controversial or indeed a panacea are discussed. Commonalities that 'miracle cures' and/or controversial therapies share are then identified through the literature, and questions proposed that parents might ask about a therapy before placing their child on any such programme. To close this chapter the development of the parent's self-advocacy skills and strong self-efficacy beliefs is discussed, and the professional's role in this process is suggested.

In the final chapter the content, responsibilities and demands of the Children and Families Bill (2013) are considered, the Local Offer described and coordinated processes for a 'once in a lifetime' assessment and the EHCP are discussed. Responsibilities at the local level are described and legislated demands made clear. Personal budgets, the appeals and mediation process and the impact on the NHS of the Special Educational Needs Reforms are outlined. How this can be to the advantage of the children and families *and* support improved shared delegation of duties for professionals is discussed.

Finally, I make the case for cooperative working arrangements in the planning and delivery of services for children and young people with special physical or mental health needs and/or educational needs. I consider that if there is to be a collaborative, effective and broad contribution from all professionals to a support team, and developmental anomalies recognized sooner rather than later, then there is a responsibility to train and prepare professionals adequately. How then can training and delivering continued professional development (CPD) be a part of policy and practice development, at the local level and beyond?

Chapter 6   **Psychosocial implications of developmental disorders**

Intended learning outcomes

At the end of this chapter you will

- be aware of a range of psychosocial issues that are the secondary impact, and frequently a consequence, of a congenital developmental disorder;
- better understand these issues, and how they impact on the child in the context of developmental theories discussed in Chapter 2;
- be able to identify what conditions prevail and impacting factors in the 'at-risk' family and develop a non-judgemental approach when offering support;
- understand why children with a developmental disorder are vulnerable in terms of internalizing or externalizing behaviour associated with mental health issues, and recognize significant key markers in each type of behaviour;
- recognize features in the developmental environment that place the child and family either 'at risk' or those that are 'protective' factors;
- understand that it is essential to promote positive social and emotional development in children and young people with a developmental disorder;
- know how to take the lead on seeking appropriate intervention or support for the child, young person or family affected by mental health issues secondary to a primary developmental condition; and
- feel competent to deliver awareness training to colleagues about social and emotional development, emotional and mental health issues and factors.

Key words (see glossary)

Adverse developmental trajectory, dissonance, ideations, pervasive disorder, somatic.

Key words (defined in the text)

Mental health disorder, mental health problem.

Introduction

It is not uncommon for any of the developmental disorders presented in this book to have a major impact on the child or young person's thoughts, feelings, relationships or behaviour, and particularly so around puberty or adolescence. But at any point developmentally, the child inevitably will notice that his or her performance or achievements are not in line with, or are different to, his or her peers. This invariably occurs when physical or cognitive limitations begin to set them apart from same-age, typically achieving children and, thus, likely to result in periods of vulnerability, when the child is 'at risk' of disengaging and either internalizing or externalizing fears or feelings of 'difference'. Children, young people and families affected by an adverse developmental trajectory experience a diverse range of needs at different times in their lives. Some of these effects as well as possible 'needs' I first identify from the perspective of the family.

The family

Depending on the nature and severity of the child's disorder, parents and siblings as well as the extended family too face a range of social, emotional, physical and even financial difficulties. If the condition presents at birth, parents and grandparents may experience a sense of loss or even grief for the child that they anticipated, and even disappointment when the child does not match the expectation. Feelings of rejection and denial are not unfamiliar. Having a child is a life changing experience, whether the firstborn or a sibling for children already in the family unit. If the new member of the family has a pervasive disorder or disability it can, by necessity, perpetually demand more emotional and physical attention, and thus leave less for significant others in the family unit. Alternatively, at the realization that the child is not developing properly marital and family tensions may ensue, and particularly so where language, motor and cognitive functions of typically developing cousins, children of friends or sibling are constantly being compared. For those whose child develops normally and then regresses at around 18–24 months there is an added loss and tension, as the child they have known begins to disappear.

The impact can have devastating consequences on the emotions of the parents, siblings and other relatives, as they experience emotional ambivalence, conflict and dissonance. There may be feelings of guilt in siblings for resenting the demands made on parents, or the focus of attention being taken so demandingly by the child with a disability or disorder. As the child develops, symptoms become more impacting on marital and sibling relationships, demands on shared family time, stress and anxiety levels are all factors that will affect all members of the family. Further stresses are centred upon getting a diagnosis of a condition. Parental resilience and family relationships are often put to the test as too frequently the assessment process can be protracted. With referral after referral the parent's advocacy role cuts more and more into 'family time'. Important time seems to be lost because of lengthy procedural delays and meanwhile the child's difficulties are becoming more and more established.

Then support and services have to be accessed and another battle can begin; plus living with uncontrollable temper tantrums or anti-social behaviour that 'excludes' the child and/or the family from events that otherwise a family could participate in. Social relationships and events are one by one gradually eliminated, and the tensions of the family can eventually become polarized to within the nuclear family unit and home environment. It is possible that the family may become closer, bonded by shared circumstances, but for many families, the reality is adults frequently are stressed, exhausted, both communication and relationships break down under the burdens imposed and cumulative factors soon begin to impact on other children in the family.

These cumulative events produce a spectrum of vulnerability at the first level for the child and family in what Bronfenbrenner (1979) described as the *micro*system (see Chapter 1). Here begins the impacting process of bidirectional influences, both away from and toward the child, and these two-way interactions operate at every system level. Parents pass on beliefs and behaviours, making the greatest impact, it is believed, on the child. But the child also affects the behaviour and beliefs of the parents. Family life is all about relationships and communication but, for example, disorders such as those on the autism spectrum are about communication challenges, misunderstood social cues and a lack of emotional understanding, and as such will inevitably impact on every relationship within the family. With a continued focus on autism spectrum as an exemplar, a summary of identified multiple tensions are evidenced below.

- With around 100,000 children with autism in the UK, approximately half a million family members are directly affected by the condition (Office of National Statistics 2005).
- Many families with a child, or children, who have autism live in poverty; to raise a child with autism it costs three times more than to raise a non-disabled or typically developing child (Sharma 2003).
- If families do not get the right support, more strain is put on the family unit. Divorce rates of parents with children who have autism is 60 per cent higher than average. A UK study showed that in families with autism, one in three were single parents (Bromley *et al.* 2004).
- Over 40 per cent of children with autism were reported as having been bullied at school (Batten *et al.* 2006).
- Young people with a disability are more likely to report being fairly or very dissatisfied with their life so far (17 per cent) than young people without a disability (7 per cent) at age 19 (DfE 2011).
- School exclusions in the UK for the child with autism are high (Ambitious about autism 2011).
- Some 71 per cent of children with autism are educated in mainstream schools in the UK; only 22 per cent of the teachers have been trained specifically in autism; 29 per cent of children with autism are in specialist provision. The amount of training given ranged from 1–4 hours; 54 per cent of all teachers in England do not feel they have received adequate training to teach children with autism (NFER 2011).

Taking this snapshot of life and living with autism, it soon becomes very apparent that mental health and well-being of all of who live within such a family unit, and not just the child with autism, are at a greater risk than others of developing mental health problems.

The child

All children and young people require, and have a right to, high-quality universal service provision, but to address the needs of the child/children and their families affected by a disorder or disability will require additional targeted support. A crisis can occur at any age or stage and may relate to health, social care or education, so what might reasonably be anticipated? This will depend on the cause, additional physical or sensory disabilities, severity of cognitive deficits or difficulties and specific neurological impairments that are presented in each individual case.

In those children and young people with a diagnosed congenital condition, psychosocial dysfunction will impact at some point developmentally. If during school days the distinctive nature of developmental disorders and the abilities and/or limitations that may impact on living and learning have not been understood in the earlier years, by the time the young person reaches adolescence manifest mental or emotional disorders may also arise, and often severely impacting on the individual's psychosocial development.

Negative outcomes can include criminal engagement as a consequence for many young people. To this end, a greater need has been identified for those employed in the Youth and Criminal Justice and Social Service agencies to receive training in recognizing 'hidden disabilities' such as ADHD or AS. The British Medical Association (BMA) has identified lack of recognition and early diagnosis of such disorders as a key factor in the rise of national crime figures in the UK, with a high percentage of crime committed by young offenders, but due in the greater part to mental health related conditions associated with developmental disorders such as ADHD www.addiss. co.uk (accessed 16 April 2013).

Behaviour issues such as 'learned helplessness' can arise when the child with a learning difficulty or disorder is unable to separate failing in one aspect of his or her life (e.g. school) from failing completely as a person (Cross and Vidyarthi 2000). This would impact on the child's self-esteem and resulting in, as a possible consequence, negative feelings of self-worth. Evidence has shown that, for example, learning problems encountered by children who have dyslexia can produce negative consequences on their self-development (Humphrey 2002, 2003; Burden and Burdett 2005) and result in major emotional, social, educational and economic repercussions (Spreen 1988). Relating this to Rotter's (1966) LoC theory (see Chapter 2) the 'external' child or learner will not only 'give up' but if the expectation of failure is high, in extremity, s/he may also develop avoidance strategies and/or behaviour issues rather than persist and strive to overcome a problem. This too 'will present with learned helplessness' (Galbraith and Alexander 2005: 29).

Lack of effort, low expectations of success and attributing success to external factors such as luck, chance or fate, these are all aligned to the concept of not only 'learned helplessness' (Maier and Seligman 1976; Peterson *et al.* 1995) but also self-efficacy (Bandura 1993) described in Chapter 2. In the learning context other influential theories are attribution and motivation (Weiner 1979) according to which the explanations that people tend to make to explain success or failure can be analysed in terms of three sets of characteristics:

- The cause of success or failure may be *internal* – we succeed or fail because of 'within-us' factors; or *external* because of factors in the environment.

- The cause of success or failure is either *stable* – the outcome for every time you perform the action the result will be the same; or *unstable* – the outcome will be different on another occasion.
- Success may be *controllable* – we believe we can change it; or *uncontrollable* – we do not believe we can easily alter or change an outcome.

(Weiner 1979)

The premise of such theories holds that people will interpret their environment in ways that maintain a positive self-image, attribute success or failure to factors within their control, be able to be autonomous, solve problems, manage emotions, experience empathy, be resilient and thus achieve psychological well-being. But if events are perceived as outside of their control, or uncontrollable, and the individual perceives their behaviour and outcomes as independent, because extrinsic forces will determine the outcome whatever, then feelings of inadequacy and hopelessness dominate. Believing this, and the individual's perception of a negative reality, produces the motivational, cognitive and emotional effects of uncontrollability or depression (Seligman 1974) and will influence future effort. Overlay such concepts onto Erikson's (1980/1994) basic conflicts in stages of psychosocial development described in Chapter 2 and tensions begin to emerge. This can include, for example, role confusion, weak sense of self and/or inferiority, weak relationships, loneliness and isolation. All of these can impact negatively on the development of the child because he or she feels 'different' or perceives themselves negatively as *unable* rather than disabled.

Physical difference and disability

Children who have a physical disability, or their physical appearance is 'different' in some way, for many reasons, are 'at risk' developmentally of feeling isolated from peers. Children with learning disabilities are more likely than their typically achieving peers (Mishna 2003) to be lonely, as are children with autism spectrum disorders (Little 2002). Particular times of vulnerability are at transition points, pre-school to kindergarten, primary school into high school; puberty and adolescence. Studies though have also shown effects of positive peer behaviour. In a secondary school setting it was found that with older classmates, when the difficulties or nature of a peer classmate's condition was explained, peer support worked well (Frederickson 2010). Schools, however, are sometimes reluctant to discuss the special needs of a pupil with their classmates because of concerns about 'labelling', although the literature has found too that such concerns have been exaggerated, and that labels can sometimes serve a protective function. Respectful and helpful relationships in adolescence, between typically developing classmates and pupils with special needs, were found to be much valued by young people, their parents and their teachers (Hudson 2010). Such relationship conditions can also become the basis of good friendships, if developed within a context of positive opportunities for interaction.

The post-16 'transition' from formal schooling to further education or training is often fraught with difficulties. Peers may be gaining independence, but the child with a disability as a young person may still require ongoing supported living. In Chapter 2, the developmental changes at puberty and adolescence outlined how the teenage years can be socially and emotionally traumatic for many typically developing children, when body image and identity of self are forming. Magnify these issues for the young person coping and living with a developmental condition or disability and the strength of impact starts to become apparent. A negative consequence of difference is bullying and it is not unusual to see bullying intensify as the child moves into teenage years. Currently in teenage cultures, cyber-bullying is on the increase, where the perpetrator does not need to deal with face-to-face verbal or psychological torment, but can use social media or mobile phone texts to attack an individual.

Adolescence is a time when traditionally young people form cliques, social clusters or gangs, and can ostracize those who are 'different' or 'outside' of the group. For the young person who has ongoing daily living challenges coping with a disability or a debilitating condition, mental health and well-being may well be 'shaky' and a time when counselling or additional support may be needed to deal with resultant mental health issues. Mental health difficulties are never caused by one factor alone, rather multiple factors, social, emotional, psychological and physical circumstances interact in different ways and manifest a different outcome for each individual. Possible risk and protective factors for children and young people with a developmental disorder are summarized in Table 6.1.

TABLE 6.1 Risk and protective factors for mental health and well-being in children and young people with a developmental disorder

Risk factors		Protective factors
Temperament, behaviour and interactional potential affected by developmental condition Low self-esteem Negative thinking	Child	Easy temperament not affected Good social and emotional skills Positive coping style, internal LoC (Rotter 1966)
Family conflict, family disintegration Inconsistent parenting styles Family viewing child in terms of 'limitations'	Family	Stable family/home environment Supportive parents and siblings/ extended family Strong family values Not seeing limitations Good advocates; parents hold positive self-efficacy beliefs.
Peer rejection, exclusionary schooling School failure, limited support or understanding of child's needs Poor home–school relationships	School	Positive inclusive school climate Equality emphasized in ethos and curriculum Needs are resources and met by the school
Late diagnosis of disorder Poor transition experiences Death in the family/emotional trauma	Life and living events	Early diagnosis and intervention Caring adults around the child in home/school/social settings Support available, but adult role models encourage traits of positivism and independence
Discrimination Isolation Lack of access to support services	Social	Support networks in the community Access to support services Strong self-identity

Mental health and well-being

Townley's (2002) distinction is made here between mental health *problems* and mental health *disorders*. Mental health *problems* are less severe, and depending on the age of the child, may include:

- feeding or eating problems;
- sleeping patterns disrupted/insomnia;
- nocturnal enuresis;
- faecal soiling with no physical cause;
- tantrums/oppositional defiance to adult authority;
- somatic pains/nausea/high temperature;
- overactive/inattentive;
- mental health *problems* may also arise as a consequence of any condition described in Chapter 4.

Mental health *disorders* are considered more severe manifestations and require greater interventions to deal with them. Symptoms may include:

- affective mood disorder/depression;
- chronic fatigue syndrome;
- anorexia/bulimia;
- post-traumatic stress disorders (PTSD);
- self-harm/ideations and/or suicide;
- any of the disorders described in Chapters 4 or 5 (e.g. ASD/WS/FAS/ADHD).

A relationship has been shown between learning difficulties and psychosocial problems (O'Brien 2006), and children with a SEN have been found to be less accepted, more vulnerable to rejection or be victims of bullying than their typically developing peers (Frederickson 2010). However, counter to this, relationships with peers have been found to be more supportive where a child has severe and obvious needs (e.g. a wheelchair user). Disabilities that impact on learning are thought to eventuate in much more than simple failure to achieve in school or acquire skills and competence, but will also include a child's susceptibility to poor adjustment and functioning in the social and emotional aspects of their development. In an unsympathetic or demoralizing environment, feelings of discouragement, lack of motivation and self-esteem suffer, and negative emotions can give rise to internalized mental health problems or depression.

Taking dyslexia as a further example, research has shown that those with poor literacy are prone to becoming disengaged from education, being excluded from school or 'drop out' before completing their formal education; are less responsive to health education; make poor well-being choices; are less able to manage chronic disorders such as asthma or diabetes; and are significantly disadvantaged in the employment market. These economic, social and personal costs of dyslexia then go some way to explain why a significantly higher proportion of young people with dyslexia are likely to attempt suicide than adolescents with normal reading age-match levels (Daniel *et al.* 2006).

In Chapter 4, ADHD features were described and showed that usually severe externalizing difficulties can often lead to early identification of problems and the provision of effective professional treatment, which can make a significant difference to children's lives. Perversely then if a child is a big enough nuisance, will something be done about it sooner rather than later?

Externalized signs of mental disorder could include any of the following:

- violent, angry or abusive attitudes;
- mood swings, temper tantrums, high state of anxiety;
- abuse of drugs or alcohol – in the older child;
- unsettled and unable to cope with day-to-day life;
- taking risks or getting into harmful/unsafe situations;
- oppositional behaviour – won't follow rules, non-compliance with adults;
- defiant and argumentative behaviour.

Exclusion from school may often be the first event identifying that a child or young person has a problem, and/or often it is the case of an undiagnosed developmental disorder such as ADHD (Sayal *et al.* 2006). It is also reported that many medical professionals feel teachers are unaware of what a condition such as ADHD is; if it really exists as a disorder, what behaviour features it presents or even realize that children with signs of ADHD behaviour should be referred. Such findings exemplify a very real need for interagency cooperation, education and training, across all frontline health care and education service providers to prevent such situations repeatedly recurring.

Signs of *internalized* disorder could include any of the following:

- withdrawn socially and emotionally, difficult peer relationships, pessimistic outlook;
- self-harming and ideations of self-harm/suicide, negative views of self-efficacy or self-competence;
- neglecting personal appearance, not sleeping, OCD, panic attacks;
- not eating/overeating, changed eating habits;
- unnatural fears/phobias or paranoia;
- nocturnal enuresis;
- neglecting school work, academic underachievement, failure to cope.

'At-risk' children such as those who are the focus here may internalize problems and suffer from mild, or in some cases more severe, depression. Such children, although less obvious than the child who externalizes or presents as a behavior 'nuisance', are possibly at a greater risk of self-harming or self-medicating through drug, alcohol or solvent abuse. The internalizer may be withdrawn and uncommunicative, and possibly overlooked in terms of intervention simply because they *do not* demand attention. They are, however, no less in need of support than the child exhibiting mental problems through externalized 'nuisance' behaviours.

A prevailing view used to be that children could not suffer from depression, or internalized anxieties, due to insufficient superego development, necessary to internalize the self-criticism thought to be necessary for the onset. This view is now refuted through research in child development (Bowlby 1980) but health professionals may find there is a general lack of understanding in the community that children, including infants and very young children, can, and do, experience mental health issues. They may even encounter limited awareness that even the very young child can also suffer from anxiety and depression, and that a child or young person's experiences with such conditions are as real and debilitating as those experienced in adulthood.

Some children may present clinically significant behaviour problems pre-school – somatic expressions of distress such as stomach pains, headaches, etc. and these frequently underpin an undiagnosed developmental disorder, but also may mask family or home conditions that are 'high risk' or even a parent(s) with learning difficulties themselves. For these children and their family the early investigation of presented, recurrent symptoms and the provision of early support or intervention may make a significant difference (DH 2004).

Depression is characterized by persistent low mood or sadness, and can affect sleep, appetite, concentration, memory and the ability to enjoy normal everyday activities that used to bring pleasure. Worst cases may require medication such as antidepressants, or psychosocial treatment or intervention through a range of options. It is also important that health care professionals involved with the treatment of children and young people with depression take time to build a supportive and collaborative relationship with the child/patient and the family. Professionals are guided here to the NICE Guidance document for clear and precise guidelines for dealing with childhood depression and I stress the point that no symptoms of depression in children or young people should be treated lightly.

Self-harming deliberately tends to be more prevalent in girls, particularly around adolescence, but this does not mean it does not occur in boys. It does, but less frequently than with girls. Around 5 per cent of all self-harm episodes referred to accident and emergency (A&E) departments are children and adolescents under 16 years of age. In this population girls outnumber boys by a ratio of 4:1 (Nadkarni *et al.* 2000). It usually involves cutting and frequently in parts of the body that are generally covered by clothing, such as the arms, and unless disclosed by the child itself is often difficult to detect. Other self-harming can also include extensive, habitual nail biting, scratching or burning flesh or, more seriously, attempted hanging. Acts of self-harming can be impulsive and secretive, and denial is often common. Self-harming can also include self-poisoning with amongst other things medication, such as Paracetamol. A relatively easy medication to obtain, most drug overdoses in the UK, US, Australia and New Zealand involve the use of Paracetamol. Its toxicity if not fatal, can also lead to long-term kidney or liver damage or even liver failure.

Substance abuse or misuse can involve the misuse of:

- alcohol;
- tobacco/cigarettes;
- illegal drugs (e.g. heroin, cocaine, ecstasy, amphetamines, LSD and cannabis);
- prescription medicines (e.g. benzodiazepines);
- non-prescription medicines (e.g. Codeine);
- volatile substances (e.g. aerosol propellants, butane, solvents and glues).

Experimentation with substances is a practice that is more widespread in teenage adolescent years and involves using what are effectively psychoactive substances or materials that when interacting with the nervous system alter perceptions, mood and behaviour. It can start out as 'fun' or to escape, to 'join in' with peers or to get through certain situations. Where a 'high' is produced the individual becomes less inhibited and often feels invincible. Studies have shown a strong connection between drug abuse and alcoholism in adults diagnosed with ADHD in childhood. As 'risk taking' is a symptom of this condition, experimenting with substances and misusing alcohol can act as a self-medication strategy for coping at stressful periods between adolescence and adulthood. It is harmful, dangerous and, if left unchecked, habitual and repeated use can, and often does, lead to addiction or death.

For further information about research in this field, the International Collaboration on ADHD and Substance Abuse (ICASA) organization is an excellent source to begin with and is available at www.adhdandsubstanceabuse.org (accessed 2 August 2013).

Anxiety is also a common mental health problem in children and young people with a learning difficulty, with heightened tendency at any age to worry, be scared or anxious about coping, or not, in everyday situations, but particularly so as they reach puberty. The child may become nervous, unable to face growing demands of school, a complex and demanding curriculum, the need for competent literacy levels and pre-examination tensions. Coping with changing attitudes and issues in the family dynamics may produce angst. For example, in a teenager struggling to master a taken-for-granted skill such as reading, or has a younger sibling who races past this young person's own reading level, feelings of inadequacy can develop; these then grow into anxieties, low self-esteem or, as previously discussed, weak self-efficacy.

Such feelings soon impact on the individual's personality, and a persistent or intense state of anxiety may develop. This will require addressing sooner rather than later if it is not to develop into a more complex or even intractable condition. In such circumstances the school nurse can help, by teaching techniques to cope with anxiety attacks. This could be a technique such as relaxation, deep breathing or rationalizing problems. Giving the child the strategies to deal with such tensions may be all that is needed.

Clear guidance on managing any of the issues discussed here can be found in the following sources:

NICE Clinical Guideline No 28 (2005) *Depression in Children and Young People: Identification and Management in Primary, Community and Secondary Care.* Downloaded from www.nice.org.uk/CG028 (accessed 1 January 2014).

NICE Clinical Guideline No 23 (2004) *Depression: Management of Depression in Primary and Secondary Care.* Downloaded from www.nice.org.uk/CG023 (accessed 1 January 2014).

CAMHS: www.camh.org.uk.

Activity 6.1: SAQs

The mother of a boy aged 14 years who has a diagnosis of ADHD has contacted you for help. Her son has been excluded from school because of his behaviour for the third time in one term, and she needs some advice.

a   Where would you go yourself for advice?
b   Where could you direct the mother for professional support?
c   How and where would you meet with the boy/access his perspective?
d   What, as a health professional, could you do?
e   What action could you initiate with the school to foster collaboration?
f   On whom could you call to form a multi-disciplinary response team to resolve this?

Intervention and support

First, in the previous chapter I made the point about seeing the child first and foremost as a person, not framed, for example, as 'autistic' or 'dyspraxic'. However adolescents, or young people with a disability, will often determine how they want to describe themselves (e.g. I have dyslexia or I am dyslexic; I have a disorder on the autism spectrum; or I am autistic). In terms of the disorder they live with, they are the experts, so counter to my earlier advice, I add that professionals from the outset should respect, and be guided by, the individual's wishes on this issue.

The second issue is a sensitive matter. The child with a disability may require additional action by professionals in terms of safeguarding, and awareness should be heightened concerning harm or abuse issues. It cannot be overstated that health professionals have a duty to follow professional guidelines for safeguarding *and* promoting the welfare of all children. But safeguarding children and young people with a disability is paramount because of their vulnerability.

Treatment and support should follow a diagnosis as soon as possible and the assessment process should lead to a list of target areas for intervention. It should include a strong psychosocial component, and usually, by necessity, involve a multi-disciplinary team of practitioners, established on a case-by-case basis, to support the child, young person or family.

The professional dealing with the young person with depression, and making the first assessment, should take into account advice given in the 'Assessing the severity of depression in primary care' document. NICE have produced some excellent tools and *Pathways* for the practitioner professional to begin initial enquiry. 'Depression in children and young people; identification and management in primary, community and secondary care' (September 2005). These are all available at www.nice.org.uk/CG28. The use of the screening tool in the CG28 NICE guidance is also recommended, and information and observations from home and school should be taken into account. Outlined below are key professionals and paraprofessionals that could offer relevant services.

Building a team around the child (TAC)

The CAF described in Chapter 1, although no longer politically a high-profile initiative, still offers a valid framework through which to collect and share information about assessed need. Decisions about the course of action needed should always take into account the child's views/family's wishes before accessing services and support. The TAC (DfE 2009) is a multi-disciplinary team of practitioners offering joined-up working and service delivery and involves:

- a lead professional to coordinate the work;
- the child and family at the centre of the process;
- a flexible multi-agency team that will change as the needs of the child change;
- a support plan to meet the needs of the child/young person;
- coordination at the point of delivery; and
- regular meetings to which the child/young person is invited to attend.

The TAC can bring together health professionals such as the HV, FNP link nurse, school or community nurse and SENCO at the child's school, as well as any paraprofessional (e.g. Teaching Assistant) working exclusively with the child. Depending on the nature of the difficulties, other professionals could include:

- GP;
- pediatrician;
- child and adolescent psychiatrist;
- clinical or educational psychologist;
- community psychiatric nurse;
- counsellor in the school setting;
- social worker;
- OT;
- physiotherapist.

The principles of collaboration and uniformity underpin a TAC and can be achieved through protocols such as:

- the needs of the child must come first;
- the family should always be present at a TAC meeting;
- meetings should follow the same format, proforma sheets are provided so the plan is consistent and understandable by all involved;
- the child's welfare is the responsibility of everyone in the TAC;
- all organizations must work together;
- the rights of the parent/carer must be considered.

CAMHS is a specialist division of the NHS to support and help young people and their families, providing help and treatment for those with emotional, behavioural and mental health difficulties. They offer guided treatment and counselling to any children and young people that are going through psychosocial or mental health issues. In particular, they offer support where needed to the children and families affected by a developmental disorder or disability.

Referral routes can be through:

- GP;
- HV;
- school nurse;
- social worker;
- youth counselling service.

Types of problems CAMHS deal with include:

- violent or angry behaviour/anger management;
- depression;
- eating difficulties/eating disorders;
- low self-esteem;
- anxiety, obsessions and compulsions, self-harming and the effects of trauma or abuse;
- sleep problems;
- more serious mental health problems such as bipolar disorder and schizophrenia.

The CAMHS website is recommended for a wide range of information for the professional, including:

- information about problems and disorders;
- support groups and organizations;
- information sheets;
- recommended books; and
- research papers.

Counselling is a way of helping the individual cope with personal issues and is offered by CAMHS, sometimes other local youth support agencies or even a school counsellor. Counsellors work with a wide range of difficulties including anxiety, depression, grief and loss, loneliness, self-esteem issues, self-injury and eating problems. It is based on a trusting relationship and allows the child or young person to express their difficulties and be guided to help deal with them. It should *not* involve judgement or advice, but should guide and support the individual towards positive coping strategies. Referral for counselling can be made through the child's GP, the school nurse or the school.

Where emotional needs are complex or protracted, different skills may be needed and the child can be referred for psychotherapy. Psychotherapists have specialist training that enables them to explore the individual's past experiences in order to help them make sense of their present life. Both counsellors and psychotherapists offer confidentiality and the professions are governed by a strict code of ethics to ensure the child or young person is in a safe environment and sensitive to the needs of those who they counsel.

CBT is a focused approach to the treatment of many types of emotional, behavioural and psychological problems. The duration and number of sessions will vary according to the problem being dealt with. It involves both cognitive therapy, focusing on an individual's pattern of thinking and behaviour therapy, which looks at actions associated with that thinking. Through this technique a skilled therapist or psychologist can help the child to overcome a wide range of emotional, psychological and behavioural problems. CBT examines all dimensions of the problem, thoughts or cognition, feelings and behaviour, as well as facing environmental situations that may be a trigger to an individual's difficulties. It is a structured, goal-orientated therapy that focuses on immediate problems as well as longer-term strategies to cope with difficulties or symptoms of anxiety as, and when, such issues recur. Skills and techniques are taught through structured therapy. These become the tools for coping that the individual can apply when overwhelmed by events or faced with new challenges or triggers that exacerbate his or her problems.

Professional skills and knowledge that are required by those at the frontline of service provision are outlined at the close of this chapter and I quote the NSF here. It makes the point that: 'All staff working with children and young people should have sufficient knowledge, training and support to promote psychological well-being of children, young people and their families' (NSF (England) Standard 9 (DH 2004)).

To do this effectively those professionals in the primary care services, including GPs, paediatricians, HVs, school nurses, social workers, teachers, juvenile justice workers, voluntary agencies and social services, need to:

- bring to the situation their specific expertise;
- ensure they have a good knowledge of how children and young people develop socially, emotionally and psychologically;
- recognize when a child or young person is experiencing difficulties, developmental delay or specific impediments to typical patterns of cognitive, social, neuromotor and emotional development;
- be able to offer, and share with support team collaborators, general advice about the primary medical, social and psychosocial impact of a developmental disorder, on children and young people, as well as be aware of vulnerability factors associated with the secondary impact on psychosocial functioning;
- know who to share information with, where to refer the child for appropriate further action and support, and the due processes to follow when looking to identify primary and secondary manifestations of specific learning or developmental disorders;
- be fully cognizant with safeguarding procedures, be aware of the vulnerability of children with a condition or disability and know they have an absolute duty, an obligation that is *not* an option, to share any anxieties they may have that concern possible abuse;
- know that better outcomes will be achieved by services working together more effectively on the frontline to meet the needs of children and young people and their families. The professional must have confidence in, and refer to, local service agreements and common assessment processes that allow for stronger interagency collaboration; and
- know how to identify those children, young people and families who are 'at risk' and/or who may need additional help, often for a wide range of support, from health, social care, education services or their community, to take a proactive role in preventing mental health and well-being problems escalating.

In Chapter 7, the focus is on meeting the needs and support from the perspective of the child. I look to identifying nurture factors and influence that impact on children and young people with a developmental condition. The network of inter-related and inter-dependent factors, and conflicting tensions, are identified through the ecological systems model introduced in Chapter 1. Evidence from children and young people with a developmental condition is given to highlight the factors they themselves consider to be important in the intervention or support they receive from professionals.

Summary

- Development theories, such as described in Chapter 2, can be extrapolated to understand how impediments, as a result of a developmental disorder, have both a primary and secondary impact for the child during the maturation process.
- The secondary impact psychosocial dysfunction is a very real consequence of a congenital developmental disorder and can place not only the child, but also the parents and family 'at risk' of psychological problems, affect their well-being and lead to mental health problems for any member of the family.
- During adolescence the self-concept becomes more complex in the young person with a developmental condition. Self-esteem contributes significantly to psychological well-being. A high self-esteem is a crucial determinant of coping ability.

- Low self-esteem, self-perception and self-efficacy beliefs are associated with loneliness, anxiety, depression and reduced well-being; manifest negative effects on atypically developing young people (e.g. ADHD/dyslexia/AS) are more likely to occur than would be expected in typically developing young people.
- In adolescence, a negative consequence of difference or disability may be bullying; at school this can be low level, teasing or tormenting, or exclusion from friendship cliques. If bullying steps up a level it can lead to isolation, withdrawal and internalized mental health problems and depression. Mental health difficulties are never caused by one single factor rather they are the result of multiple factors that interact in different ways.
- A family approach may be needed where a family is 'at risk' due to a pattern of vulnerability. Families of disabled children may experience high levels of unmet need, isolation and stress as a result of a range of social, economic and environmental factors.
- A lack of support, or unmet needs, from appropriate services for the child and their family can result in further isolation and family tensions.
- As a lead health professional in a multi-agency team of support for the child, and for the family, there is a need for interagency professionals to receive training to increase awareness of developmental disorders that are described in Chapters 4 and 5, particularly in dealing with mental health and psychosocial issues that are a secondary impact of a disorder.

Signposts to further information and guidance

NICE has developed mental health guidelines in collaboration with the National Collaborating Centre for Mental Health (NCCMH) and different products are associated with particular mental health topics. NICE guidelines are published online from www.nice.org.uk. The NCCMH publish full guidelines as a book and accompanying CD-ROM, produced by the British Psychological Society and the Royal College of Psychiatrists.

NCCMH (2005). *Depression in Children and Young People: Identification and Management in Primary, Community and Secondary Care*. Leicester and London, British Psychological Society and Royal College of Psychiatrists.

NCCMH (2011). *Common Mental Health Disorders: Identification and Pathways to Care*. Leicester and London, British Psychological Society and Royal College of Psychiatrists.

NICE (2004). *Eating Disorders: Core Interventions in the Treatment and Management of Anorexia Nervosa, Bulimia Nervosa and Related Eating Disorders*. NICE clinical guideline CG9. Downloaded from www.nice/org.uk/CG009 (accessed 2 January 2014).

NICE (2004). Self-Harm: The Short-term Physical and Psychological Management and Secondary Prevention of Self-harm in Primary and Secondary Care. NICE clinical guideline CG16. Downloaded from www.nice.org.uk/CG016 (accessed 2 January 2014).

NICE (2004). *Anxiety: Management of Anxiety (Panic Disorder, with or without Agoraphobia, and Generalized Anxiety Disorder) in Primary, Secondary and Community Care*. NICE clinical guideline CG23. Available at www.nice.org.uk/CG023 (accessed 2 January 2014).

NICE (2004). *Core Interventions in the Treatment of Obsessive-Compulsive Disorder (OCD) and Body Dysmorphic Disorder (BDD)*. NICE clinical guideline CG31. Downloaded from www.nice.org.uk/cg31 (accessed 23 December 2013).

NICE (2005). *Depression in Children and Young People: Identification and Management in Primary, Community and Secondary Care*. NICE clinical guideline CG28. Downloaded from www.nice.org.uk/CG28 (accessed 1 January 2014).

NICE (2007). *Interventions to Reduce Substance Misuse Among Vulnerable Young People Public Health Guidance (PH4)*. Downloaded from www.nice.org.uk/PHI004 (accessed 2 January 2014).

NICE (2011). *Common Mental Health Identification and Pathways to Care*. NICE clinical guideline CG123. Downloaded from www.nice.org.uk/CG123 (accessed 1 January 2014).

RCN (2009). *Mental Health in Children and Young People. An RCN Toolkit for Nurses who are not Mental Health Specialists*. London, Royal College of Nursing. Downloaded from www.rcn.org.uk/__data/assets/pdf_file/0003/235299/003311.pdf (accessed 1 January 2014).

Chapter 7   **Working with the child or young person**

Intended learning outcomes

At the end of this chapter you will

- understand, through the context of an ecological framework, how health professionals delivering a universal child health and support service are both compelled and constrained by opposing interests;
- appreciate how policies and resources can shift according to political forces and changing systems in society, while also acknowledging that former policy planning is still of value in present and future practices;
- understand the tensions, and conflict of interest, between meeting the needs of children with a developmental condition, SEN and/or disability and the allocation of funds available;
- understand the difference between listening and hearing experiences and views expressed by clients who are children and young people; be aware of strategies through which to access their views and to enhance professional interactional skills that facilitate a broad body of information from the child; and
- be aware of international trends and formulaic models used to allocate the funding of services and developmental health and learning support for the child and family.

Key words (defined in the text)

Social capital, therapeutic encounter.

Introduction

First in this chapter the social or nurturing bioecological environment introduced in Chapter 1 (Bronfenbrenner 1989/1992, 1994) is used to frame enquiry. The model recognizes that each individual, as well as the family as a unit, is significantly affected by interactions in the overlapping contextual levels, systems or environment. The ever-changing variables within these systems and factors that impact and obstruct early diagnosis and deliver intervention are examined. The universal health visiting service in the UK is about enabling children and families to have the best start in life, but where the child has an adverse developmental trajectory, meeting additional support needs can mean the frontline professional is constantly faced with opposing tensions. Some such tensions and conflicts of interest within systems in England are identified here.

Policy and its effect on events that occur outside of the family are examined, particularly in events within *macro*systems, and institutional patterns in the culture, economy and political governance are discussed. These have a profound effect on the quality and nature of relationships and actions within the family; these I explore as possible constraints to efficiently address the needs of the child, or children, with a developmental disorder where they present with additional needs.

The Bronfenbrenner (1994: 40) conception of time, the *chrono*system, is considered to 'encompass change or consistency over time, not only in the characteristics of the person but also of the environment in which that person lives'. Change as a response to time and its impact on the child, policy and practice are examined here. The focus then shifts to the views and experiences of children and young people, to *what* they are saying about their specific needs; how they perceive problems; and *how* they are heard. The distinction is made between 'hearing' and 'listening' to the child. Findings from studies with young people and strategies for accessing children's views and experiences are presented.

To close this chapter the issue of meeting the cost of universal health, care and SEN or disabilities is then discussed, and international trends in funding models and resource allocation are then explored; their relevance I link to the Children and Families Bill (2013).

Exploring bidirectional influences through the 'systems' model

In the previous three chapters, developmental disorders were presented, and associated affective needs explored, at both the primary level, i.e. the immediate impact of a condition (Chapters 4 and 5) and the secondary level, where psychosocial functioning is compromised (Chapter 6). The need to identify and resourcefully support children, young people and their families in dealing with both levels was also highlighted. Emphasized throughout is the need for early diagnosis and intervention, both crucial factors in setting the stage for positive longer-term outcomes for the child's future.

It is now recognized that early child development, even without the presence of a congenital developmental disorder, is a key social determinant of health and health inequalities. It is also a critical period for intervention and this I link to the underpinning principles of the universal health visiting service. The service remit in England, and other UK countries, is around enabling children and families to have the best start in life and, in particular, targeting those families with additional needs. Political forces, through progressive universal services, also signal a strong commitment to support families and young children, provide some support for all, but more for those with greater affective need (e.g. in children with conditions that have been described). This message has been reinforced through the myriad of initiatives, guidelines and policy documentation summarized in Chapter 1 and referenced throughout this book.

Universal services such as health and social welfare are invariably the closest contact to a child post-natal, next to the mother, and there is an expectation that the mother and health professional will work together to prevent problems occurring, or to improve outcomes for the child. In reality this premise may not necessarily be supported and the ecological systems framework allows us to consider negative assumptions and adverse tensions in the nurturing environment.

Bronfenbrenner's (1994) paradigm takes into account linkages and processes between two or more settings that contain the developing child, and across the settings that do not contain the developing child but where events immediately affect him or her. What needs to be understood is all systems are interrelated with bidirectional influences passing to and from the child. The ecological model is utilized here to explore patterns of activities, social roles and interpersonal relations experienced in the nurturing environment by the developing child, and structures closest to him or her. This includes the family, the community or the setting wherein the child is placed, and health and social care agencies wherein relationships and interactions occur that will affect the child, both around and in the wider social structures.

Tensions around the child

To undertake a holistic assessment of the neonate the HV comes to the family with an unusual degree of universal acceptance. Their 'longstanding entrée to the home of all parents from birth to school entry' (UKPHA 2009: 15) means the HV is usually successful in gaining acceptance by families across society. However, there is also a small percentage of families with whom service providers find it difficult to engage at any stage (Carbone *et al.* 2004). The relationship between the family and external support services will vary according to the values held by the parent, the family and the professionals who are delivering the health and social services, but who are also making both subjective and professional value judgements.

In the UK, health promotion specialists are increasingly aware that health-related behaviours are shaped, and constrained, by a range of social and community contexts and I use Putnam's (2000) conceptualization of 'social capital' here as a means to explain. In this theory 'social capital' refers to social networks and interpersonal relationships with central components at the individual level being trust, reciprocity, trustworthiness, community and 'civic virtue' (ibid.: 19). Civic virtue refers to civic engagement where members actively participate in a trusting community; where individuals actively involve themselves, know each other and have a trustful and helpful relationship.

The premise here is that 'social capital' operates at different levels and socialness, the medium through which social capital operates, can be anywhere along a spectrum from weak through interconnected and durable to strong. In order to achieve a strong community with high social capital, there has to be trust, reciprocity and mutuality between members of that community. For the individual on the outer edge of a community, who may hold negative views and perceptions about systems, in this example the public health system, and does *not* engage with those involved with delivering frontline health services for whatever reason, there will be a degree of reticence about engaging in the services that are on offer.

The HV then may not always be welcome, but may be perceived as someone in authority that is invasive, even a threat, and parents might be reluctant to accept advice or collaborate with the very professionals who are there to support them. Frontline service providers such as the HV have a duty to safeguard and protect children in their care, and a parent, or another member of the family, may perceive this aspect of their role as threatening or judgemental. Thus from the outset the professional's intentions may be distrusted.

Family-held values and attitudes are passed intergenerationally or nurtured in the culture or overarching characteristics of subculture within the *macro*system wherein the child is placed, and consequently can be in conflict with those who are offering the support. It may require a sensitive and intuitive approach to break down barriers that could impede developmental surveillance and jeopardize early identification of a within-child disorder or developmental condition.

It has been said earlier that parents are often the first to suspect their child may have a developmental problem, and their concerns should always be taken seriously. They may not have understood the significance of their observations, but they are generally very efficient at detecting that something is amiss, but the relationship between the professional and the parent needs a 'safe space' where they can share 'concerns'. The *meso*system that Bronfenbrenner (1994) theorized represents such an interactional setting or space. Here processes are characterized as connecting linkages and processes, two-way communication, participation, decision-making and joint involvement across two or more systems that contain the developing child. The child is not directly involved, but the interrelationship between the adults will, in due process, affect the outcomes for the child.

In this broader setting then, events can take place that are crucial in terms of the child's outcomes. Should the health care professional fail to listen to, or take, parents' views seriously, early detection and the referral system can break down. The active involvement of parents in the assessment of young children with developmental disabilities is a well-established principle in early childhood intervention services. Such partnerships with families can be seen as the cornerstone of developmental assessments (Miller and Hanft 1999) and health professionals are thus in a prime position to observe and identify deviating developmental patterns or 'at-risk' indicators in the child that may alert them to early symptoms of a specific developmental disorder.

Moving then to when parent(s) have concerns, Sayal (2006) identified four stages as periods where parents seek help to allay concerns about developmental anomalies in their child, and these are:

a   parental perception of problems;
b   raising concerns with primary care services;
c   recognition of problems within primary care; and
d   referral to, or use of, specialist health care services.

Here further tensions can be identified. It could be argued that any of these four stages not only give access to further help but they can also act as filters that may prevent children being referred for specialist help, and would depend very much on several variables. For example (a) *parental perception*, the crucial pre- and post-natal developmental phase viewed at the *micro* level, identifies the genetic and environmental influences, the face-to-face relationships and experience, the family and the linkages that take place between significant others that share the settings wherein the child is placed and, importantly, that interact in the setting that the child is born into. The efficacy of the parent's judgement about their child's development could, it is argued, be better than the health professional. For example, they can provide two broad types of data: clinical information and behaviour observations, and can describe their child's past and current functioning. Interestingly too, parental concern for their child's development has also been shown to be an accurate indicator of true developmental problems, regardless of differences in the parent's education and child-rearing experience (Baird *et al.* 2001). It should not, however, be presumed that this is so in all cases.

Although generally the parent(s) does perceive a developmental problem (a), for many different reasons, they may not. The parent(s) may avoid (b) *raising concerns*, because they are in 'denial'; have learning difficulties themselves; are already on the 'at-risk' register because of safeguarding issues; or have personal, cultural or religious reasons for not wanting their child referred. Viewed through processes at the *meso* level the impact on two-way communication and participation in decisions between the parents, family and professionals may thus be inhibited. The parent and/or family may well resist professional attempts to refer their child for further assessment, and although hopefully this would be the exception rather than the norm, professionals should thus avoid holding assumptions about such a course of action.

Recognition of a problem within primary care (c) may also occur later rather than sooner. From the professional's perspective, as developmental theories presented (see Chapter 2) have shown, child development is not a regular transition from one stage to another. Children develop at different rates, and although professionally the frontline service provider may recognize a developmental delay, at what stage does it indicate something more? Each of the disorders presented have also shown that symptoms each condition present are not necessarily indicative of one straightforward diagnosis, change as the child develops and, with a few exceptions (e.g. WS/RS), are rarely identified by blood or gene pathology. Which brings us to the issue of referral (d) *referral to, or use of, specialist health care services* and here again frontline service providers can act as gatekeepers to the next level of service.

Change over time

I draw first on the Bronfenbrenner (1994) concept of the *chrono*system, the final system parameter in the model that extends the developmental environment into a third dimension. This encompasses change or consistency over time in personal characteristics, but also in the child's developmental environment. Two emerging factors are considered here, although there are many more.

First, if developmentally the child is changing *and* so too is the nature of the symptoms the child presents, how sure then can the health care professional be that a referral to a specialist clinician should be made? What if there was insufficient evidence for concern, a lack of key indicators present in the child or the development profile of the child is only marginally outside of the 'normal' parameters described in such measures as the SGS II? These examples stress not only the value of public health initiatives, and strategic plans to monitor and promote child health and well-being across all agencies, but also the need for high standards of professional training to ensure health professionals have the skills to recognize when something developmentally is 'amiss'.

Second, the 'gatekeeper' role may present a conflict of interests for the professional. Children and young people with a developmental disorder frequently experience a mix of educational, health and social disadvantage. In the UK in this the twenty-first century, and despite shifting political and organizational influences that have traversed through theorized *macro* levels, evidence would suggest that current services fail to detect and/or address *all* of the children that have a congenital developmental disorder. Examples are shown in England, where children that are on the autism spectrum, and some with CP, are missing out and not being identified until late on (Evidence 2011). Nor, as the Bercow Report (2008) showed, has the need for well-qualified speech therapists across many regions of the UK been addressed.

It is well understood that any support or intervention should produce a desired outcome, effectively and efficiently, while incurring wherever possible the least cost, low cost *or even no cost*. The latter criteria you would never find overtly declared in any health, social care or education policy document, but at the risk of appearing facetious, I see creative, expedient and efficient use of funding as not only guiding principles but also the greatest challenge in most public services.

I emphasize the point here that frontline health services are constantly faced with a fiscal dilemma. The issue of funding I discuss later in this chapter, in particular the model legislated for in the Children and Families Bill (2013), i.e. a 'personal budget' or 'direct payment' model to give the young person and their family control over purchasing special needs support services. First though, I discuss the need for professionals to both listen and hear what the child, as a client and consumer, is saying, and strategies that aid the process of accessing the child's perspective.

The child as a client: listening to and 'hearing' the child

Earlier the position of the child and children's rights embedded in law, policy and practice was made clear (Chapter 1). The point was also made that 'not only should we take account of children's views but we also have a moral obligation to enable [children] to articulate their views as effectively as possible' (Cooper 1993: 129). Gersch (1996) too posits pragmatic reasoning, that views from children be considered as they have information to contribute about themselves, where the adult may too easily assume that the young person's views are exactly the same as their own. There is a need for health professionals to create the potential for children and young people to have their own ideas and views heard and understood, and should look to evidence-based research in health to explore methods that have successfully generated different information from the young person's perspective (Morrow 2001b).

There has been a surge of interest in the need for children's voices and opinions to be heard, stimulated by national and international changes in the legal rights of children. The focus here is on accessing the child's views. Children and young people have been consulted about issues affecting them socially (Morrow 2001a: 255), educationally (Flutter and Ruddock 2004) and concerning the provision of health services (La Valle *et al.* 2012). A children's health and health education study, grounded in the 'child's voice' paradigm, found children not only had views but they could also express them very well (Scratchley 2003). Moreover, adults participating in the study were surprised when they realized the extent of the issues about health that children were both grappling with and thinking about (ibid.: iii).

The point of view of the child then, previously ignored perhaps because of pre-sumed incompetence, has been challenged by social science research (Morss 1991), as has the point made elsewhere that children have been invisible and voiceless objects of concern and not understood as competent autonomous persons who have a point of view (Smith and Taylor 2000). The voices of those with SEN have shown that children have a great deal of important information to contribute about them-selves (Lewis and Lindsay 2000; Humphrey and Mullins 2002), a view supported elsewhere by adolescents who had dyslexia (Hudson 2010). This study found young people very capable of producing analytical and constructive observations, and could react responsibly to the task of identifying factors that could impede, or further, their own learning.

Communicating and successful interactions with children and young people are important to ensure appropriate assessment, management and intervention in support-ing their specific needs. It is 'no longer acceptable for organizations to view individuals with learning disabilities as passive recipients of services; they must instead be seen as active partners' (DH 2001: 51). A study of views from clients using CAMHS services, and who were children with learning disabilities (Boyden *et al.* 2013), advocated that in both policy formation and the support that is offered, frontline services working with children and young people need to consider the following points:

- offer a welcoming approach;
- communicate at a level appropriate for the client;
- evaluate the impact of the work your service carries out; and
- identify from the clients themselves the difficulties they encountered.

This study advocated the use of photographs and/or visual aids, or novel interactive tools such as books, pictures and play dough, telling a story or drawing, to access the child's perspective. Imagery and metaphors were also considered a useful device through which to explain feelings, e.g. anger, such as an erupting volcano or as a calming strategy by imagining being under the sea (ibid.: 57).

It has been suggested that nurses, when assessing and working with young peo-ple, need to find a way of interacting that is somewhere between having a chat and doing therapy (Cooper and Glasper 2001). Further, that nurses first need to break down personal barriers to effective psychosocial assessment. Describing the concept of a 'therapeutic encounter' as a 'dynamic and sensitive interaction between what is "known" [professional knowledge] and what is "yet to be known" [the patient's story]', Cooper and Glasper (ibid.: 35) suggest also that two key elements must be present for this interaction to be productive.

The first element is the capacity of the nurse to have an internal conversation, to engage with both personal beliefs and 'tribal stories'. This internal dialogue should be reflexive and take account of their position in relation to the young person's 'tribal' story. The tribal story allows the nurse to enter into the world of the other and, through an internal narrative, to internally assimilate what the world of the young person is like in terms of attitudes, systems and beliefs. The second element is the nurse's 'therapeutic style', or the aspects of their interpersonal communication that can enhance therapeutic properties.

Listening to children

The HVs and school nurses have an important role in the early assessment and delivery of effective intervention. Routine but stringent ethical procedures should *always* be followed and particularly so if working with children and young people with learning disabilities. Certain ethical tensions therefore need to be considered when accessing any child's view, particularly surrounding issues of ethics, consent and confidentiality. These cannot, nor should not, be disregarded. The child, prior to being interviewed, has the right to know what information you are looking for, and what you are going to do with that information. At the initial stages of a meeting too much information can be as confusing as too little, and promises made about confidentiality must be carefully judged.

At the outset it is necessary that the professional does not generate anxiety in the child, and children have the right *at all times* to know that some forms of information, once disclosed, must be reported further, particularly where there is a risk in terms of child protection. Be sure then that before giving any assurances or making any commitment to confidentiality these factors have been thought out.

Disabled children, and particularly those with communication disorders, may require alternative language support systems (e.g. British Sign Language; Makaton; AAC methods). Where the child has very limited vocabulary or understanding, or the ability to communicate is impaired by complex needs, professionals have a responsibility to support communication to ensure the child fully understands and effectively makes their view or perceptions known. For children with more complex needs the Hearing the Child Service provided by Barnardo's will provide resources and other communication tools specific to the child's needs; and will also act as an intermediary if required to facilitate communication between the professional and the child (www.barnardos.org.uk/seenandheard.htm (accessed 28 July 2013)).

Also to facilitate the child's voice being heard the Children's Society offers advocacy services to children and young people with disabilities, in particular for disabled children placed away from home. In addition they support and promote advocacy and family participation in any decision-making processes. The society will also offer expertise in supporting children who have significant SLCN (www.childrenssociety.org.uk (accessed 19 July 2013)).

Problems can arise with babies and young children that are unable to express themselves in words, or with older children who may feel uncomfortable speaking about their problems of difficulties in front of other family members or in certain environments. How these can be circumvented will depend very much on the specific case and the innovative skills of the professional. Some basic techniques to guide the interview process with children and young people with adverse developmental trajectories are given below.

Practical guidance for interviewing children and young people

- Make the environment for the interview a safe environment.
- Draw up a schedule for the interview, sequence your questions but be flexible.

- Avoid too rigid a structure in your questioning framework. Do not let the framework take control of the conversation away from the child.
- Construct an 'about me' sheet: I like/I don't like; I have/I don't have; I can/I cannot, etc.
- Ask about pets/siblings/something s/he may have made or won.
- Allow the child to talk about something with which s/he is familiar and/or has some expertise (e.g. computer programme; climbing/balancing; solving puzzles; *Thomas the Tank Engine*).
- Avoid interrupting the child if they are talking about seemingly irrelevant topics – some of what they are saying may be very relevant.
- Allow the child to draw a picture and talk about what they are drawing. Place the focus on the drawing and this will make the interaction less intense.
- If the child withdraws or becomes uncomfortable, turn the focus back on to an activity to 'keep the flow' of the interview going.
- Avoid uncomfortable silences. Have a distracter at hand in case (e.g. puppet, small puzzle, toy) age appropriate to the child.
- Try to give some control to the child and if they introduce new subject areas, follow their lead. Return to your interview schedule when appropriate.
- A low-key casual conversational approach may sometimes be the best route to take.
- Provide the child with an array of questioning formats. This is especially helpful if the child is not particularly verbal or responsive.
- Use puppets or dolls to present questions or as a medium that will allow the child to respond.
- Have a range of activities at hand, change the activity if boredom or tiredness becomes apparent.
- Use different questioning formats, age appropriate, to help keep the child engaged and interested.
- With babies and young children use direct observation.

Techniques to 'listen to the child'

Active listening involves:

- observing and reading non-verbal behaviour, body language, facial expressions, etc.;
- listening *and* understanding the message they are trying to convey;
- listening to the whole person, within the context of settings within social systems;
- accepting as valid the child's feelings and views of themselves; and
- putting aside personal interfering variables (e.g. bias or prejudice).

Impediments to effective listening could include:

- a mismatch of value systems between the professional and the child or young person;
- being judgemental or pejorative, making unfavourable comparisons between the child client and perhaps the professional's own child;
- allowing professional knowledge to cloud your judgements;

- not hearing the right message because of listening to facts rather than feelings and emotions being expressed; and
- being too distracted by other work issues, uncomfortable/distracted by the time constraints.

Successful interactions with children require the child to recognize, understand and express emotions and feelings appropriately, whether in happiness, fear, anxiety, distress, love or loneliness. Emotional literacy will not only allow them to express these emotions respectfully to others when necessary, but also understand emotions, and that these emotions can change. I return to this topic again in Chapter 8, where I look at how emotional literacy can be developed by those working in the TAC.

What children said in a study by the National Children's Bureau (La Valle *et al.* 2012) about health provision is summarized in Table 7.1 and shows that children clearly identified both negative and positive factors in their experience.

TABLE 7.1 Positive and negative features identified by children using health services

Negative	Positive
Communication: lack of explanations, not communicating with them, not being involved with decisions affecting their care. Doctors did not speak directly to them, or speak in a language they could understand when they DID speak to them	Effective communication at an appropriate level Provide accessible information in a format that is accessible to the age/maturity of the child
No choice: not being consulted or asked their opinion about their treatment	Informed and involved: involved in the management of their treatment
Lack of respect, being treated as 'stupid', being ignored, being patronized. Lack of privacy. Not taken seriously	Respect: offering acceptance and empathy; privacy and confidentiality; dignity and respect for feelings
Stress: too few opportunities to describe/express their discomfort. Not always listened to	Active participation in their care; more involvement; evidence that their involvement had made a contribution to change
Service provision: the way health services were delivered could be a barrier to achieving aspirations. Lack of early interventions	More support in the home and family support; providing family members with training and guidance from professionals
Multi-agency care: felt 'in limbo' not knowing which agency to go to; school nurse not accessible	Person-centred, multi-agency planning: more involved with a named keyworker
Not child-friendly providers of care: mental health 'stigmatizing' conditions, lack of information about mental health issues. Too judgemental; felt 'blamed' and 'it was my own fault'	Clinical competence but able to relate to children through flexible and responsive support Importance of relationships with practitioners

Source: adapted from La Valle *et al.* (2012).

In a family support group for young people with a diagnosis of AS, young people aged between 11 and 19 years were asked the question 'what would you like friends, teachers, nurses and people in the community to know and understand about AS?' Their responses were overwhelmingly detailed but the sample given below I considered poignant, pertinent and worth noting. The young people referred to those who are *not* on the autism spectrum as NT.

- No two people on the spectrum are the same. AS has different manifestations in different people but our brains do operate differently to NTs. We understand things but in a different way to NT people. You think us odd but we have to learn what 'odd' is and what you think is 'odd' about us.
- Please don't expect me to look you in the eye, I find that very difficult to do so if you want me to look you in the eye when you are talking to me, I cannot. I am not being rude or obtuse I just find it too uncomfortable to do.
- We are very sensitive to background noise, e.g. a lawnmower outside the window, chairs scraping, other children talking, humming lights or computers, these can all distract us.
- We're like diesel engines compared to petrol engines. Please don't try to change me or cure me. Yes we have some special needs and may need help to function like NT kids.
- I get very anxious, may flap my hands or do certain behaviour over and over again. This gives me a feeling of security that sometimes we haven't got, like in an unfamiliar place or situation. It may distress you to see me do it, but it is more distressing to me if you try and stop me from doing it.
- We don't understand facial expressions but we can learn what expressions mean. We need to be taught and it takes time.
- I have a disability but I am not incompetent. We are not idiots so please don't treat us in a condescending manner; understand we work hard at some things that NT kids do naturally and easily.
- I don't learn social skills easily, they are never automatic and can learn them over time, but also, unless someone points out what is expected of me, where and when I will forget and appear rude. I don't mean to be but I don't always know that I am being rude. I don't have many friends but please don't force me to mix with groups. I cannot always cope with being included.
- Routine is important to us, we need routine as it gives our life some order and security. When routines change we need time to prepare and adjust to it so will be unsettled for a while.
- If I'm misbehaving badly, or oddly, it may mean I am overwhelmed with too much sensory information. When I can't cope I can go into a meltdown and have to escape *immediately*. I don't run away because of you, or to be defiant, I *have* to get away from situations sometimes *urgently*.
- Please allow me a quiet space if I am anxious or stressed. Please don't touch me, some AS people don't mind being touched and held but some cannot tolerate touching or physical contact.
- I don't respond well to shouting or ranting. If you are angry with me, tell me so but quietly and rationally.

Activity 7.1: Reflective practice

Begin by identifying what you think could be barriers to good practice in placing the child at the centre of a plan to support the child with an ASD and his/her family. How first would you engage the child and what methods could be devised to access his/her views? Building a multi-professional team and sharing of responsibility for the child or young person with such a disorder or disability requires many personal and professional skills. Identify what skills would be to the advantage of a multi-agency programme. What features would you think were essential to make this shared model of provision work? What professional qualities do you think would be valued within such a model? How would you begin to involve the child or young person or the parents and educate them in terms of *their* expertise and the *value* of their knowledge? How could cross-profession, CPD make a positive contribution to the quality and level of support for the child with such an adverse developmental trajectory as manifest in autism? What support would you see as most beneficial for the family particularly where there are older or younger siblings?

To conclude, in general adults, and particularly professional adults in service organizations, develop policies and practices for, and on behalf of, children and young people. But there is increasing evidence that consulting with the clients of 'child-friendly' services, the children themselves make a valuable contribution in the planning *and* evaluation of policies that directly affect them. By listening to children, adults can align their actions with children's rights. Importantly, even very young children can tell adults quite a lot *if* they are asked the right questions, and allowed to respond in a manner that is age appropriate and 'user friendly'. It has been said elsewhere that the new image of children emphasizes three key ideas: that even young children can construct valid meanings about the world and their place in it; know the world in alternative (not 'inferior') ways to adults; and their perspectives and insights can help adults to understand their experiences better (MacNaughton *et al.* 2004).

Crucially remember too that when interacting with young people, closely observe and be aware of different cues. Hear what the child is saying, in both verbal and non-verbal language, and develop best practice of listening carefully and hearing also what it is they may *not* be saying.

The thorny issue of economics is discussed next. Sharing and allocating finite resources present many ethical dilemmas and professional tensions. International formulae and models of funding that give context to such issues are the focus here.

Meeting the cost: funding and resource allocation

Resources have to be allocated to meet all needs, and within the extent of finite resources, funds have to be allocated to meet a) the needs of the child; b) the family; and c) the legal demands that specify a child's rights and entitlements. Professionals in health and education not only have to constantly face opposing tensions, but are also constrained in terms of meeting their professional demands. Universal health visiting is understood as 'a proactive, universal service that provides a platform from which to reach out to individuals and vulnerable groups, taking into account their dynamics and needs, and reducing inequalities in health' (UKPHA 2009: 6).

Contextualizing services within exosystems, delivering a service to improve social health and well-being, specifically children and families, in the face of so much change and fiscal restraint is a challenge, with positive and negative consequences. For the family whose child has additional needs, decisions within systems occur on a daily basis, interrelated between two or more settings that do not contain the child, but which in their outcome will almost certainly affect the child.

A lack of funding allocated to the referral system, or a lack of a suitably qualified or a specialist professional to whom the child can be referred, may slow down processes, causing not only an 'in-system' delay in identification and diagnosis, but also the application of an appropriate intervention programme or treatment. Factors in, and across, systems then can be both supporting or constraining, with the interconnections between the family and the professional, and the outcomes for the child, very much depending on favourable factors being operant. Is this then almost comparable to a favourable alignment of the planets perhaps?

With regards to the dimension of time, however, public initiatives, strategic plans to promote health and well-being and standards of professional training have moved forward, developed in response to fluctuations at the *macro* level, both politically and economically. The global economy suffered a major collapse around 2008 that produced an ongoing period of global economic instability. Post 2010 and following the UK general election, a shift in governing dynamics occurred. This brought about new policies and guidelines that reflected the position of the Coalition Government (Conservative and Liberal). Since then change and adaptation has occurred, including budget cuts, cuts in public services and reshaping of the NHS. Reverberating influences and events, way beyond the control of individuals, impacted broadly and effected global and local changes across all systems.

In the UK, drastic reductions made in funds available for public services, inevitably, meant reductions in the level of services that could be provided. The larger *macro*system, society and policy, may not interact directly with families, but their influence and the consequences make a significant impact on them. High unemployment and families coping with redundancy, loss of an income, change in parent employment roles, all add to stress levels and challenge coping systems of family members. Factor that onto the family that has a child (or children) presenting with developmental anomalies and the stress is compounded further.

Numerous policies and initiatives developed in the decade from 2000–2010, some mentioned in earlier chapters, have been revised, jettisoned, renamed and/or updated. Additionally new policies and legislation have come on line. Prevailing political and socio-economic forces may shape services and support but do not necessarily bring about *great* changes. Rather, changes in the structure of support systems are more subtle than revolutionary.

One change though that *is* significant and making an impact in both design and delivery of services is the Children and Families Bill (2013) and I expand on this further in Chapter 9; but crucial here is the move from the old system of assessing and managing SEN through mainly education systems, to health, to ensure that the health service 'plays a greater part in delivering all of the support that each individual child with special educational needs and disabilities has' (TSO 2012: 15).

Central to this administration is how funding is to be allocated and managed with a move to 'personal budgets' and 'direct payments' that place the parent and/or young person in control of funds, to secure and maintain services, or particular provision specified for the child or young person with an EHCP. The EHCP is a single plan following an integrated single assessment approach, and that reflects the needs of the child from birth to 25 years of age. Local authorities are exploring different ways of administration and the model that evolves will depend upon the outcome of pilot trials.

International funding allocation formulae

In the absence of one UK model to describe, I draw here on international trends and formula funding that operate elsewhere, and that address the funding issues for specific needs required by children with affective needs. It is not necessary to get too bogged down with the mechanics and application, rather this overview provides examples through which to better understand how they can, and do, work elsewhere. SEN funding mechanisms in the US (Parrish and Alberts 2009), Australia and New Zealand (Mitchell 2010) are described.

Census-based models in Australia allocate funds on the basis of the number of pupils with certain 'weighted' characteristics such as socio-economic status or type and degree of disability. This makes financing of special education independent of classification and placement decisions, and removes the 'perverse incentives' (ibid. 83) for over-identifying students as having a disability. In the US, census-based funds are allocated on the amount of students enrolled in a school, a formula detached from any count of special need. Again this reduces 'fiscal incentives' (Parrish and Alberts 2009: 9) that may be associated with increased identification of certain types of disability or SEN.

Discretionary funding models provide separate funds for SEN purposes. They 'enable individual schools to make decisions about the type of services and programmes to support' (Mitchell 2010: 87). This may be a percentage of the school total budget and used to purchase services, support or teacher aid for the pupil needing specialist services or intensive support, and mostly applied where a child has complex high needs or disability that is severe. In the US, the term 'pupil weight' (Parrish and Alberts 2009: 9) describes a similar model, where funds are allocated per pupil and is based on some characteristics of the special education student.

Categorical funding models allocate additional funds to pupils identified with a learning or physiological disability/SEN, the amount being based on the level or degree/type of the disability or need, which equates to the 'pupil weights' model in the US. The advantage of this is that it recognizes difference in cost according to need, *but* it may provide an incentive to over-identify those with disabilities. In Australia, funds might be allocated to the child's school or to the parents to meet the needs of the child. The advantage being that funds are transferable and if the child moves to another school the funds are portable and thus move with the child.

Voucher-based funding models make a direct public payment to the parent to cover the child's private or public costs. The value of the voucher will depend on the nature of the need or disability, and may be paid to the parent or school on behalf of the parent. This model aims to increase parental choice and to promote competition between schools 'in order to increase the quality of educational services' (Mitchell 2010: 87).

Percentage reimbursement in the US is based on actual district special education spending and eligible expenses determined by the state. The 'district' is then reimbursed for a set percentage of the total amount. The disadvantage is, according to Parrish and Alberts, the 'burdensome accounting' (2009: 9) and the advantage being the percentage of reimbursed accounts for varied categories of disability.

Actual costs funds are, according to Mitchell (2010: 87), allocated on the basis of the actual costs involved in providing special education services. Total funds are allocated to schools on the basis of the number of students meeting the definition of mild and/or more severe multiple disabilities (ibid.: 88). As with categorical and census-based funding models, the total amount of funding is based on the student numbers with SEN in any school.

In conclusion then, funding of special education, learning needs and disabilities is a complex affair and an ideal single funding model seems to be elusive. All models presented have strengths and weaknesses, as well as positive and negative outcomes that will affect individuals differently, thus a combination of funding models would seem to be needed. From a purely economic viewpoint, allocating resources to where they will do the most good would appear to be most efficient, but would that also be discriminatory? Indeed doesn't that premise also involve making a value judgement about what the 'most good' is and for whom? Where conditions for accessing support are stringent and criteria-based there is always going to be the child who is 'just outside' the set parameters, and finding any one system to meet all needs is always going to be a challenge to the policy makers.

To address this, policy makers looking at models of funding should perhaps aim to ensure that they address the following factors:

- early identification;
- school and health policies that support pupil functioning from pre-school into the inclusive school setting;
- it offers intensive education support for those struggling with learning in schools;
- flexible funds to accommodate children with complex needs;
- avoid undue incentives and disincentives;
- be allocated coherently through systems policies;
- directed to approaches for which, in any audit of effectiveness of support, there is evidence of effectiveness in improving outcomes for the child and the family;
- be transparent and equitable and show a clear pathway to spending and outcomes;
- ensure arrangements are accountable, can be monitored and outcomes can be measured.

In Chapter 8, a case study that demonstrates successful multi-professional collaboration is presented in the SA. I then look at the vulnerability of parents with a child or children that have an adverse developmental trajectory, and the role of the professional as an advisor, or advocate, for 'fads' or 'miracle cures'. The chapter closes with a look at models of parent advocacy.

Summary

- A model such as the developmental environment employed here allows for identification of both positive and negative factors that impact on delivering a universal health service. It can reveal limitations and forces that act against the best interests of the child and the family, conflicts that professionals have to deal with and the interrelationship between past, present and future models of service provision.

- Past and present policies when contextualized alongside future policies can be acknowledged in the shaping of what happens next. Evolving legislative processes and future models of service provision are inextricably linked to those operating in other developed countries and subjected to the same global fluctuations.

- Social and/or interactional tensions may compromise initial meetings with the parent(s) for many different reasons that may not be related to the here and now. Concepts such as 'social capital' and 'socialness' are useful to contextualize a family's relationship with structures in society.

- Methodologies for including children's voices and enabling their active participation in assessment and intervention programmes should be given full consideration at the outset; augmenting strategies for accessing the child's perspective may require the professional to devise novel and/or alternative options and include innovative technology if necessary.

- It is important to remember that 'listening' is not the same as 'hearing', and 'being safe' is not the same as feeling safe. The subtleties between them are very significant when interacting with children and young people who have additional needs that their specific condition may incur.

- Decisions made about who and what support can be offered have to be based on judgements that are fair and can be overtly justified. Models of funding presented here have shown there is no single 'best' funding model; every model has weaknesses, incentives and disincentives that will affect the children differentially.

- Means of allocating resources continues to challenge policy makers around the world; fiscal funds at the national level will always be outstripped by demand.

- Proposed personal budgets/direct payments to parents will require professionals to give objective, informed guidance to parents and the family about what services or therapies are appropriate to their child's needs, and what allied professional services need to be purchased.

- Resources should be directed to approaches that, through evidence-based studies, have been shown to be effective in improving outcomes for children and young people with manifest difficulties from a specific developmental difficulty.

- Policy should allocate resources where they will be of the greatest advantage, and models of allocation should take this into account when criteria are being decided. Resources should be allocated through a consistent, objective and logical process.

Chapter 8

Development of multi-agency policy: supporting the parents

Intended learning outcomes

At the end of this chapter you will

- understand through a case study how responsibilities can be shared, and the need for parents, while supported by professionals, to play an active part in addressing identified needs;
- understand that change doesn't instantly happen but a change in attitude, practice, policy and commitment to professional partnerships can achieve positive changes in service provision and support for children and families;
- acknowledge that scant funds or limited resources should not be a limiting factor in implementing change;
- understand, and reason, why some parents are difficult to engage, or accept, professional support in the identification of need and subsequent intervention put in place to support their child;
- know and understand why parent vulnerability may lead them towards non-scientific, non-bona-fide therapies to address their child's needs;
- be able to draw rational, independent conclusions about 'fad therapies', 'miracle cures' or alternative treatments; conduct your own rigorous, analytical and critical approach to information, and present a critically balanced opinion if asked; and
- acknowledge that support is most effective when underpinned by the promotion of supported family involvement and a culture of self-advocacy training for parents.

Key words (defined in the text)

Antioxidants, cerebellar-vestibular dysfunction, chelation, cognitive dissonance, containment, salicylates.

Introduction

Achieving collaboration is the focus of this chapter and here I describe a joint venture between psychology, psychotherapy and health visiting that also involves the mother *and* father. The example here, presented in a case study, shows how policy can successfully promote 'change' and deliever cost-effective practice. The theoretical principles of the Solihull Approach (SA) translate into the consistent working practices I describe. The appeal of the model as an instrument to engage whole families including fathers, and the effectiveness, viewed from the perspective of both parents and professionals, is corroborated through the research studies and literature presented here. Next, an overview of treatment and intervention 'fads' and 'miracle cures' is presented and, for the health professional who is working with vulnerable parents, guidance is offered about evaluating 'treatments' and 'therapies' that make claims about positive outcomes for children that have an adverse developmental trajectory or a developmental disorder. The chapter closes with a look at how community institutions can enhance the parent's self-efficacy, and capacity to themselves to seek help for their children's difficulties, through advocacy agencies and by engaging the whole family, including fathers.

The Solihull Approach (SA): a case study

Background

It has been stressed that developmental disorders, such as those described, invariably present developmental anomalies of which all professionals involved with young children need to be aware, in particular HVs and adults working in childcare, playgroups, day care and kindergarten. There is a need to not only bring together a range of expertise to aid diagnosis, but also a need to further the knowledge base and training of professionals such as those in disciplines of psychology, medicine, optometry, physiotherapy, occupational and speech therapy and nursing. Universal services such as health, education and social welfare are often the first, and closest, points of contact to a child or young person, and an approach that is multi-agency and person-centred is advocated for a holistic appraisal of additional needs. Support from a range of services can be advantageous, but so too is the need for parents to play an active part in addressing identified needs, while being supported by professionals. The SA has successfully incorporated many of the demands outlined above and not only exemplifies good practice in terms of collaboration, but also demonstrates how change of practice 'across services' has been successfully developed first, in one local area, and then widely adopted elsewhere. Developed in 1996 this service delivery model involved Hazel Douglas, who led a joint venture between HVs, child psychotherapists and clinical psychologists in CAMHS, and was developed in Solihull, UK. Initial motivation was to support HVs in their work with families with children with feeding, sleeping, toileting and behaviour difficulties. Its strength however has been its adaptability and this case study will show how it has evolved, and continues to cover an ever-widening range of professionals, from different agencies, to work with families to manage a range of health and social issues.

The SA Parenting Group further developed the model

- to create an effective parenting programme by focusing on the parent–child relationships and promoting a reflective style of parenting;

- to provide a group that helps parents with children from 0–18 years;
- to promote the use of shared language between professionals;
- to reduce problematic behaviour in children and affect parental anxiety; and
- to provide an evidenced-based parenting programme that facilitates joint working between agencies supported by a robust and cost-effective training model.

A pilot evaluation of the approach found that over the course of the ten-week parent group training, parental anxiety and child behaviour problems improved significantly, and changes were both measurable and correlated positively on the Becks Anxiety Inventory (BAI) and a Child Behaviour Check List (CBCL) (Bateson *et al.* 2008).

Theoretical framework for the original SA project evolved not from new theory but from a combination of three different theoretical ideas and extension of them to practice. The constituent concepts are

- containment (psychoanalytic concept; Bion 1959);
- reciprocity (child development concept; Brazelton *et al.* 1974); and
- behaviour management (behaviourism concept; Skinner 1938).

Bion (1959) saw the concept of containment as central in the role of the mother in the developmental trajectory of the infant. Arising from the traditions of psychoanalytical theory, deriving from Freud's work, it describes the process whereby the parent is able to support the child in the process of dealing with intense feelings of emotions and anxiety, as opposed to being overwhelmed by them. Implicit is the notion that it helps to develop the child's capacity to think.

Applying this to the work of the HV, it was found that the HV served a containment function, containing the anxiety and overwhelming feelings of the parent, and restoring in them 'the ability to think' (Douglas and Ginty 2001: 222). This empowered the parents to solve the problems for themselves. Containment then, summed up, is where a person receives and understands the emotional communication of another, calmly and without being overwhelmed by it, and communicates this 'calm' state back to the other person. In parenting, it helps the parent to think about their child, to relate and to cope with anxiety and emotion. It also helps the parent to process some 'old' emotions so that the parent can relate to the actual child in front of them, not to a 'projection' of a child.

Reciprocity is the basic unit of an interaction in a dyad, or an interaction between two persons, and is present in all relationships. In child development theory, it describes the early mother–infant interaction, and the process whereby mother and infant develop their interaction, turn taking, to reciprocate communication. HVs are able to observe and deduce the level and quality of reciprocity in mother–child interactions. Where reciprocity is lacking, it may indicate that active interactions are compromised and negative effects for babies of mothers who suffer from post-natal depression have been observed (Tronick 1997). Reciprocity, then, describes the sophisticated interaction between a baby and an adult where both are involved in the initiation, regulation and termination of the interaction. Reciprocity is not a concept applicable solely to infant interactions. It can also be used to describe, and observe, the quality of interactions within all relationships. In parenting though, it enables parents and their child to relate, tunes parents in to think about their baby, increases their awareness of their child's needs, provides a focus and a language for feeding back to parents about the interaction and is crucial in the development of parenting skills (Douglas and Ginty 2001).

Behaviour management has evolved in psychology from behaviourist theory, and behaviour management is part of the ordinary process of normal development and parenting. Parents in well-functioning families work together and use reinforcement all the time for desired behaviour, punishing undesired behaviour and, additionally, placing reasonable boundaries on the child to control behaviour. They encourage the child with attention and other rewards. Parents teach their child self-control and, gradually, the child becomes able to internalize both the restraints and the satisfactions for him/herself, thus enabling the child to participate and function adequately in society.

In the SA parenting support model, the HV helps the family by observing if, or where, this process has broken down, and by making suggestions that when the parents feel sufficiently confident, they can put some changes into their parenting practice. The approach has been found to reduce parent anxiety while significantly improving child behavioural problems (Bateson *et al.* 2008). Further, parent feedback following instruction through a SA parenting group in the understanding of a child's behaviour showed that 'understanding' preceded change (Johnson and Wilson 2012) and helped parents to relax and share experiences. Such a finding fits within social learning theory that presumes we learn from others in different ways, and it takes time, change doesn't instantly happen.

Research and evaluations

The body of literature from evidence-based research and articles shows the efficacy of the SA is growing. Studies from the perspective of the parent (Douglas and Ginty 2001; Douglas and Brennan 2004; Maunders *et al.* 2007; Johnson and Wilson 2012); parents of children with complex neurodevelopmental difficulties (Williams and Newell 2012); HV practitioners (Whitehead and Douglas 2005; Milford *et al.* 2006; Stephanopoulo *et al.* 2011); and other professionals (Lowenhoff 2004) have, to date, been published, and ongoing research is also evaluating the father's perspective (Alan Dolan, Warwick University). In this 'Father's Project' (Dolan 2013), small study positive comments made by fathers post-programme confirm changed father–child interactions, and a difference in the engagement with their child(ren) as corroborated through the following quotes.

> Yeah it's definitely changed. Without a doubt. It's massively different now... My parenting style's absolutely nothing like it was... I'd never dream of raising my voice now... That's one thing I've definitely learnt... I've learnt voice tones... That's what it's all about is talking and explaining... We're a lot more bonded. Without a shadow of a doubt.
>
> (Robert, 42, son aged one year, daughter aged 19 years)

> This whole thing's about being in tune. I've definitely seen development there. Nothing stresses me anymore... I feel so relaxed... I've never felt more kind of relaxed... It's a lovely environment at home. It's really helped.
>
> (Michael, 30, son aged 11 months)

It has opened my eyes in a lot of aspects, in a lot of ways, to deal with my children in a better way... I ain't shouted... if they've done something wrong, I ain't shouted at 'hem. I've just sat them down and explained... Before I'd probably have shouted at 'em. And then took them in the bedroom and shut the door. I don't do that now... It's a lot calmer and my kids seem a lot happier.

(Gavin, 30, son aged two years, daughter aged five years)

Qualitative research has provided insights into changed perceptions and parenting behaviour; and explored concepts of trust, empathy and understanding in parent–HV relationships (Maunders *et al.* 2007). Quantitative studies have also shown measurable correlations between the programme and positive outcomes (Milford *et al.* 2006; Bateson *et al.* 2008). Improved confidence has been shown in HVs and family support workers (Moore *et al.* 2013) and findings reported include changed emotions about their work and service (Whitehead and Douglas 2005). Although a small sample study, grounded theory elicited themes that showed HVs had a greater ability to focus more on emotions, were more reflective about their practices, had increased job satisfaction, improved consistency in procedures and improved relations with colleagues in the service.

The value of the approach to a range of professionals including HVs, nursery nurses, school nurses, SS workers and school counsellors as well as cost effectiveness of training and changed practice has also been evaluated (Lowenhoff 2004). Findings also demonstrated significant improvements in a range of outcomes, for both children and families, without having to invest in major new resources, apart from the initial expense of providing the training. A key factor in the success of the SA model has also been recognized as resting on good leadership, the crucial role of managerial support, supervision and consultation in implementing the training in practice (Moore *et al.* 2013).

To summarize, effected positive changes in HV practices include:

- consistency in practice;
- better time management – able to better plan family contact in terms of time and resources;
- case management time reduced;
- increase in follow up after initial assessments;
- enhanced understanding of the role of containment and reciprocity;
- improved confidence in their own approach, skills and practice;
- more holistic assessments at first took longer, but quality of assessments improved;
- follow-up times reduced;
- contact HV time decreased; and
- positive outcomes achieved more quickly.

Projects and developments derived from the SA model include:

- an integrative model for training across agencies (Douglas and Rheeston 2009);
- the issue of containment for HV anxieties and the role of supervision;
- information leaflets for parents in language that is at an appropriate level;
- targeted home visiting interventions (Walker *et al.* 2008);
- Masculine and Fathering Identities Project (Alan Dolan, University of Warwick);

- fast-track HV referrals to CAMHS;
- HV referrals supporting the HV with CAMHS;
- a whole school approach developed (Douglas 2011);
- resource packs for professionals to use in their work with families to deliver training or run a parenting group (The First Five Years and The School Years);
- a trainer's training manual;
- reducing burnout and stress; the effectiveness of clinical supervision (Wallbank and Hatton 2011);
- the Solihull Approach Parenting Facilitators Resource pack – one-day training for parent group management; and
- the Solihull Approach Antenatal Resource Pack and Parenting Group.

As shown earlier, the influence of early experience (Chapter 2) on brain architecture is crucial in the early years of life. It determines future emotional, intellectual and physical development. Early bonding and secure attachments with those close to them lead to the development of empathy, trust and well-being. But as seen in previous chapters, disorders may observably impact not only on the attachment process but also on sensory, motor, social, emotional and communication development.

This psychotherapeutic approach, based on concepts of containment, reciprocity and behaviour management, allows this model to focus on more than just supporting experience for parents. Project groups of HVs, child psychologists and child psychotherapists, as well as professionals from other agencies, have also had an input, contributing their expertise when, and if, necessary (Douglas and Ginty 2001). Thus the approach now embraces an ever-widening field of need, has been adopted by many local commissioning services groups nationally and internationally, and is aligned to NICE guidance – the Parent Training/Education programme in the management of children with conduct disorders. (The NICE reference relates to the implementation of NICE guidance: TA102-NICE TA102 Parent Training, Solihull Approach information website. Downloaded from www.solihullapproachparenting.com (accessed 2 January 2014).

Fad therapies, miracle cures and parent vulnerability: some general characteristics

The purpose here is not to dwell on the merits, or otherwise, of any one particular treatment or intervention that claims to remediate a specific disorder, rather I present a sample of treatments that when first popularized, were considered radical, controversial or indeed a panacea; some I briefly mention elsewhere (Chapters 4 and 5). Neurophysiologic therapies of patterning, cerebellar-vestibular dysfunction, sensory integrative therapy and a chemical therapy used to treat autism, chelation, are presented. Dietary modifications and food additive theory follows, and commonalities of 'miracle cures' and controversial therapies are then identified. Questions that professionals and parents should ask about a therapy are offered, and to close this discussion, the role of the professional in advising or advocating controversial treatments with vulnerable parents, and the child, are discussed.

There are many unconventional approaches to address learning disabilities and the point I've made elsewhere is that the field of learning disabilities per se is littered with dead ends, false starts, pseudo-science and fads (Stanovich 1999). A 'fad' refers to a practice or interest followed for a time with zeal, and commonly manifests as exercise programmes and/or diets (Braganza and Ozuah 2005). Some therapies may be based on pseudo-science, others on bad science, but if developmental learning difficulties disrupt family dynamics, or cause anxiety or frustration, in this situation an alternative treatment or management approach can be especially appealing.

A 'miracle cure' will often be promoted intensely, glowingly, uncritically, with intimate personal testimonies and endorsements, sometimes from celebrities. It is therefore understandable that for many vulnerable parents, this style of marketing could be considered to constitute evidence of a treatment's efficacy. It is also often the case that when evidence repeatedly shows such programmes to be ineffective in the longer term, it has done little, or nothing, to stem the flow of such programmes onto the market. How then can parents and carers judge if an intervention is effective when it is first heard about in the media? Bishop (2008) identifies specific questions to ask of a new treatment that would seem to be particularly poignant for both parents and health professionals when considering involvement in any such therapy. I make the point, first, that the therapies presented are examples, and that none of the cited therapies here are under criticism.

Neurophysiological patterning: Neural Organizational Technique (NOT)

Underpinning theory of 'patterning' first proposed in the 1960s (Doman and Delacato 1968) follows the principle of the child's failure to pass properly through a sequence of developmental stages in mobility, language and competence in the domains of manual dexterity, visual, tactile and auditory skills. The hypothesis makes explicit that children must achieve full development at each level and without deviating from the normal sequence (Gottlieb 1989). Incomplete development reflects poor neurological organization and deficits may manifest as learning disabilities and behavioural problems. Treatments encompassed in patterning therapy programmes include passive movements, sensory stimulation and re-breathing of expired air (claimed to stimulate cerebral blood flow). Various diet restrictions of fluid, salt and sugar claim to decrease cerebrospinal fluid (CSF) production and cortical irritability. Treatment involved repetitive activities using specific muscle patterns in the sequence that the child should have learned *if* development had been 'normal', e.g. rolling over, sitting, crawling and walking. The programme aims to correct the disorganization in the CNS and is described in the literature as reaching all of the stimuli normally provided by the child's environment but with such intensity and frequency that, ultimately, a response will be drawn from the corresponding motor systems (Doman and Delacato 1968).

Aligned to NOT and such conditions as CP or severe brain damage, is the notion that imposing patterns of passive movement can produce behaviour or activities, that a developmental unimpaired brain would have produced. The literature does not throw up much in the way of published research that investigated the treatment as successful for learning disabilities, and concerns have been expressed about the treatment. These came through policy statements of both the American Academy of Paediatrics (AAP) and the American Academy for Cerebral Palsy and Developmental Medicine (AACPDM) who, after reviewing all the relevant literature, found patterning treatment offers no special merit and 'offers false hopes' (Gottlieb 1989: 252).

The therapy protocol in the case of CP requires numerous volunteers to assist with delivery of the treatment regime, demands rigid time schedules and strict adherence to the programme. The therapy became less popular in the late 1980s but current interventions are available that are based on the concepts inherent in patterning.

Sacro-craniopathy-mobilization therapy

Craniopathy is the art and science of osteopathy and chiropractice and deals with the relationship of the cranial structure, CSF and body mechanics. A sac-like membrane called the dural membrane covers the brain and spinal cord and contains CSF. The CSF, created in the ventricles in the brain, acts as a cushion, protecting this delicate mechanism, transporting nutrition and removing waste products. It provides an ideal medium for essential nerve energy condition. The CSF flow or circulation is essential for many reasons and is gently pulsed around by breathing and cardiovascular functions. Impediments to this 'flow' may be caused by the bones of the skull being misaligned, as a result of birth trauma or injury, and results in CSF being unable to flow easily. If misaligned they interfere with the pulse-like waves and gentle 'mobilization' realigns them, allowing the brain to function optimally. Cranio-sacral therapy is presumed to serve as an effective way to remove blocks to the efficient motion of CSF. Claims made are that this will result in enhanced motion of the CSF, producing overall body energy. It is attributed to the authors (Ferreri and Wainwright 1984) as an intervention therapy for dyslexia in *Breakthrough for Dyslexia and Learning Disabilities*, now out of print. Underpinning theory posits that learning disabilities are caused by damage to two specific cranial bones, the sphenoid and the temporal bones. Theory speculates that learning disabilities occur because the displacement of the sphenoid and temporal bones cause neurological problems by creating unequal pressure areas on the brain. Treatment involves specific body manipulations to correct the difficulty with identified cranial faults.

The authors reported that most learning disabled individuals responded in a positive way in one to three treatments and remained clear of symptoms on a schedule of reinforcement visits; adding that once the neurological and structural corrections are made, the person is cured and able to learn what he or she was not able to learn before. Having achieved this level, the next phase of treatment is referred to as 'catch up'. This refers to what the individual must learn that he or she did not learn before the correction. Remedial tutoring is necessary. If the child does not make progress with tutoring, the authors suggest that the cranial bones may have slipped back out of position and further treatment is required.

Chelation and autism spectrum disorders

Many methods of intervention and treatment have been, and continue to be, associated with an ASD. Special diets and elimination diets are discussed later but links have also been made between autism, heavy metals and chemicals 'within-child'. Chelation therapy is one 'advocated' treatment through which to deal with this 'poisoning'. It involves the introduction of chemicals, either orally or intravenously, which then bind to poisonous metals such as mercury, arsenic and lead so they can be excreted. This is an approved treatment for heavy metal poisoning but it can be dangerous, and is *not* approved for use in treating autism. However this does not mean to say the practice is not being used. Analysis of five chelation studies in the US showed that none provided any certainty that any benefits that were shown to have occurred in the children were due to chelation itself, and not just the developmental maturation that had occurred over a time span (Hannaford 2013). Chelation is a good example of why a health warning should always be given about *non*-evidenced-based treatments, that have *not* undergone rigorous, well-designed scientific studies, and peer reviewed in respected professional journals.

Cerebellar-vestibular dysfunction therapies

Underpinning theory for cerebellar-vestibular dysfunction implicates the vestibular system in learning disabilities and, particularly, impacts on children's mastery of reading and written language. A causal relationship is drawn between vestibular disorders and poor academic performance and the impact of motor defects and underlying organic brain deficits. There is a theorized belief that the dysfunction can be treated by controlling sensory-motor behaviour and that, in turn, will influence neurosensory integration.

Activities considered important in correcting behaviour and/or deficits include vestibular, postural and tactile stimulation (Ayres 1972b; Levinson 1980) and have been linked to theories of cerebellar-vestibular dysfunction in dyslexia. Disturbances in the complex interaction of inner ear function, coordination of eye–head movements, ocular fixation, tracking and fixation are ultimately reflected as specific reading disorders.

Therapy proposes the use of anti-motion sickness medication to correct the vestibular dysfunction. Associated symptoms are described as poor postural coordination, poor balance, poor spatial orientation and nystagmus, and the rapid and involuntary movement of the eyeball. Following evaluation for the dysfunction, therapeutic intervention had popularity in some countries and attracted research to establish empirical standards. Claims suggested sensory integration therapy had a significant effect on perceptual processing dysfunction and academic achievement. However unresolved issues and contradictory data influenced a recommendation that caution should be observed when considering participation in these therapies (Gottlieb 1989).

Dietary modification: food additives

Probably the most well-known theories of the 1970s implicated food additives, flavouring and colours in learning difficulties and hyperactive behaviours. Theory suggested that food additives could trigger these behaviours in susceptible children (Feingold 1975). At a time of changing diets and greater consumption of processed foods and ready-meals, this linked the increasing prevalence of children presenting with developmental behavioural disorders to the increased use of synthetic colouring and flavouring. The theory was that removing food with some additives (e.g. artificial colours, preservatives, synthetic antioxidants, etc.) from a child's diet would result in improvements to both behaviour and learning. Feingold therapy involves dietary control, the elimination or reduction of artificial food contaminants to which the child may have reacted and, reportedly, it had alleviated some symptoms quite dramatically in a number of cases. Numerous clinical studies that examined the outcome or response to dietary modification empirically tested the claims of the Feingold hypothesis. For some professionals, and a large number of parents, the treatment continues to have considerable appeal, and adaptations have been made as the therapy has evolved over the years. Underpinning theory views a food allergy as an immune system response and, by identifying and eliminating something from the child's diet that is an irritant or trigger, in the longer term, it can have a beneficial effect on the child's behaviour. Elimination or allergy diets are used to isolate food allergies or food sensitivity.

The science underpinning food additives has vindicated some of the issues. Research has shown that a strictly supervised elimination diet may be a valuable instrument in testing young children with ADHD, as to whether specific dietary factors are contributing to the manifestation of the disorder (Pelsser *et al.* 2008). Studies from Australia (Dengate and Ruben 2002) and the UK produced evidence that certain food additives can influence hyperactive behaviour (Bateman *et al.* 2004). From overall findings in 2008, the UK Food Standards Agency (FSA) requested a ban on the use of some well-known artificial colours namely Tartrazine, Quinoline Yellow, Sunset Yellow, Carmoisine, Ponceau Red, Allura Red and sodium benzoate. Subsequently, the European Union (EU) ruled that food labelling in EU member countries must, by law, carry a warning that states 'may have an adverse effect on activity and attention in children'.

A current focus in the additives debate is on naturally occurring salicylates in food. Based on his evidence drawn from 1,200 cases, in which the phenomenon was considered to be associated with learning and behavioural disorders, Feingold suggested that many hyperactive children are sensitive to these. Foods high in natural salicylates, similar to a component of aspirin, include strawberries, kiwifruit, avocados, sultanas and other dried fruits, citrus, pineapple, broccoli, pizza toppings, tomato sauce, olive oil and tea. Information about low-chemical elimination diets free of additives and low in salicylates, as well as food intolerances, can be found in the books and/or website of Sue Dengate (http://fedup.com.au).

In terms of autism, special diets and elimination diets are often implicated in potential 'cure' claims even though there are no known advantages for children with autism, and concern has been expressed that such diets may cause the child to get inadequate nutrition. Gluten-free casein-free (GFCF) diets are promoted by those that support 'leaky-gut' claims in autism, underpinning the theory that 'leaky-guts' allow opiods to escape into the bloodstream and then travel to the brain and cause autistic behaviours. However there is no evidence available for this claim. Further, children on the GFCF diet have been found to have lower bone density than controls that could, over time, lead to osteoporosis (Hannaford 2013). Gastro-intestinal problems and exclusionary diets have been mentioned earlier (see Chapter 5) and are built on a premise that a yeast form, candida albicans, may be a causal factor in autism, or exacerbate behaviour and health problems in those who have an ASD.

Antifungal drugs and supplements sometimes combined with a yeast-free diet is a treatment option, although research has yet to establish the efficacy of such treatments. Parents have reported behaviour changes as a response to elimination diets (Pennesi and Klein 2012) but caution should be applied when considering the results of this relatively small study (n=387). Data was generated through an online survey, with no control study, and with parents reporting changed behaviour with a reduction in ASD core symptoms. However these parents had been expecting a change to occur, and this could have caused a placebo effect, or influenced what they perceived as a positive result of dietary changes.

Commonalities of 'miracle cures' and/or controversial therapies: a critical approach

The novel nature of many controversial therapies or treatments is often given a high media profile when it is first placed in the public domain. Newspapers, magazines, radio and television carry claims of dramatic improvements or cures from those who have undertaken such therapies. 'Cures' are often evidenced through testimonials and anecdotal data and such claims are generally more convincing to the general public than scientific empirical studies reported in academic journals. It has been said elsewhere that controversial therapies share common shortcomings (Golden 1984), some of which include:

- a theoretical basis not always consistent with principles established by scientific rigour;
- treatment is liberally recommended for a broad spectrum of developmental and behaviour disorders;
- often promulgated as 'non-harmful';
- controlled studies fail to replicate claims made; and
- generally promotes management in isolation – often procedures protected by a 'commercially sensitive' caveat.

A scientific approach to enquiry requires a critical approach to the examination of claims made about the intervention and for 'a product or program to be considered a cure for disease, there are several desiderata or criteria to be met' (Stephenson and Wheldall 2008: 68). Using a medical model that applies equally well to an education or health intervention, I paraphrase their five criteria here.

1   The disease must be operationalized specifically to assure objective diagnosis.
2   Cause of the disease must be established unequivocally and located conceptually within, and building on, known science while adopting 'the most parsimonious explanation that fits the available evidence'.
3   Proposed treatment should be objectively operationalized to ensure subsequent replication *and* needs to be shown to directly affect the known cause of the disease.
4   The treatment must be shown reliably to reduce or eradicate the symptoms of the disease in persons who have been reliably shown to have the disease.
5   Others, external to the original research group, must readily and frequently replicate the demonstration of efficacy.

Smith (as cited in Stephenson and Wheldall 2008) summarizes characteristics of what are termed pseudo-scientific interventions as:

- claims of cures and reporting important sounding but vague outcomes;
- evidence from uncontrolled studies; or
- the more subjective data sources as found in anecdotal testimonials.

The underlying theory may be in conflict with accepted knowledge in a given field of study and often describes core deficits that can be corrected, and thus result in, improvements in a given array of areas. General characteristics of both controversial and acceptable therapies identified and adapted from those described elsewhere (Gottlieb 1989) are summarized in Table 8.1.

TABLE 8.1 Characteristics of controversial and acceptable therapies

Characteristic	Controversial therapies	Acceptable therapies
Theoretical construct	Weak underlying hypothesis	Constructed from established neurological, biochemical or educational theories
Therapy focus	Makes claims of cures for a diverse range of disabilities	Designed to address a specific disorder
Side-effects	Usually non-invasive, non-harmful, sometimes a 'natural' intervention	Recognized side-effects, patient alerted to possible side-effects
Claims of efficacy	Popularized by media/testimonials/cases	Peer reviewed in professional journals; design conforms to stringent, scientific methodology
Therapy design	Usually used as a single therapy; inadequacy of compliance as cause of failure	Usually adjunct with other treatments, e.g. special education/counselling/medication
Replication of data	Other studies fail to replicate the claims made	Results are comparable in other replicated studies
Lay 'untrained' group response	Promoted/endorsed by lay groups as panacea or cure	No strong endorsement for the treatment from lay groups
Professional response	Reluctant to recommend therapy. May accept the approach if other therapies fail to improve symptoms. May agree to trial period of participation with reviews of progress	Will recommend and monitor standard therapy. Awareness of shortcomings considered, patient informed. No guarantee given that a positive outcome will result

Source: adapted from Gottlieb (1989: 254).

Vulnerable parents: questions to ask about a treatment

In their combined efforts to help children overcome the barriers to development and learning, parents, health professionals and teachers are all partners. When parents express an interest in exploring a controversial therapy or a miracle cure, professional opinion is often sought either to advocate or challenge its stated aims or claims. As a professional, parents may expect from you effective, impartial counselling that may influence judgements about signing up their child to a therapy or treatment. In such circumstances there is a need for the professional to appreciate the parents' vulnerability. Often as a result of disappointment and growing frustration waiting for the system to address their child's special or additional needs, parents may enthusiastically embrace controversial therapies for their child. It could be to avoid the psychosocial stresses of their child 'being different', or because such a therapy may appear to provide an alternative solution, a quick fix or a 'cure'. As such their vulnerability is frequently the precursor for signing up their child for treatment that may be costly and limited in its alleged benefits.

As Bishop (2008) explained, there is a human tendency to think that something that has taken time, effort or money is worthwhile, and the concept of cognitive dissonance, a phenomenon in psychology, serves to explain this rationalizing or justification process in humans. We have a tendency to filter out information that conflicts with what we already believe, in an effort to ignore that information and reinforce one's beliefs. When after a specific treatment, another person tells us how much better they feel, and if that person is someone we respect, the message has greater potency than any table or graph. Thus public endorsement from a celebrity or a respected professional is a powerful advocate and will carry weight for parents at the decision-making stage.

The questions that Bishop (ibid.) posed to ask about a treatment are considered here to be appropriate for both parents and professionals alike.

- Is the theory scientifically plausible?
- Does evidence for efficacy go beyond testimonials?
- Have studies been done with groups for whom the treatment is recommended?
- Is there evidence that gains are due to the treatment?
- Are the costs reasonable relative to the benefits?

It is not the professional's place to tell parents what they should, or should not, do in terms of trying new treatments, but these guidelines, borrowed from science, offer a sensible benchmark by which to make a judgement about a programme's efficacy. This is particularly important when there are commercial interests at stake, where it can be hard for a layperson to evaluate the claims that are being made, and where there may be a financial investment to be made by the parents. To bring to a close this discussion, speaking specifically about autism, author Michael Fitzpatrick, whose son James is autistic, gives a valuable and poignant insight into parent vulnerability. He describes the impotence he felt watching James regress at 18 months, after he had been developing normally, adding:

> Doctors will say they don't know what causes it and there's nothing you can do about it – two things that are difficult to live with. The need to 'do something' can be overwhelming. And then someone else comes along and says your doctor is useless, that they know what caused it, and that you can do something about it. One reason special diets are so popular, despite being unproven, is that they give parents something to do on a daily basis.
>
> (Hannaford 2013: 29)

Recommended further reading

Wilson, B. A., F. Gracey, J. Evans and A. Bateman (2009). *Neuropsychological Rehabilitation: Theory, Models, Therapy and Outcome*. Cambridge, Cambridge University Press.

Activity 8.1: Internet and online search

Find websites that direct parents to reliable information and advocacy support in the following situations.

1   A parent thinks her two-year-old son may have an autism spectrum disorder.
2   A mother thinks the school are failing to identify the needs of her daughter age seven years who is struggling to acquire fluent literacy skills.
3   A paediatrician has finally told a parent that her son, aged 18 months, has been diagnosed as having WS.
4   The parents of a girl age two years refuse to let their child receive a measles, mumps and rubella (MMR) vaccination because they have heard it is linked to autism.
5   George age nine years has severe difficulty concentrating for any significant length of time. Mother thinks he has ADHD.
6   Because he is recognized on a psychologist report as 'high functioning', an LA has refused to put resources into school to support Tom age 12 years who has a diagnosis of AS.
7   The mother of Luke age ten years is diagnosed as having ADHD co-morbid with dyslexia and has heard about a new exercise regime programme that can 'cure' both dyslexia and ADHD.
8   The parents of Emma age nine years and diagnosed with ASD have heard about a diet and something called 'leaky gut' that may be causing some of her problems.
9   Jake age 11 years had a diagnosis of ADHD and his parents think he needs Ritalin. They are worried how Ritalin will affect him and if it is an addictive drug.

Parent advocacy and support

Fundamentally health professionals should try to achieve being an aid to problem solving rather than the solution, or solver, of problems. Ideally relationships should aim to form a vital social and emotional foundation to shared responsibility, and frontline service providers need to develop the parent's self-advocacy skills and strong self-efficacy beliefs. This, with support, will empower them to take control and make positive decisions about their child's needs.

Typically a family advocacy approach may take the form of a campaign for an under-represented group, to change or challenge policy, in the belief that collectively they have the potential to enhance support or provision for those children or families that have a need that is not being addressed. In this model, individuals and families can be seen as bringing an influence to bear that may change systems at a macro level.

Others may approach advocacy through a non-partisan body, but a goal to advance what they deem most desirable for the family and child's specific needs, looking at options available and often in the light of their own value system. Such a body could be seen in the Independent Parental Special Education Advice (IPSEA) organization, which helps parents access provision or support for specific needs by taking up the mantle on behalf of parents and children if they are not in a position to do so themselves.

Advocacy is most beneficial to families when it encourages families to be involved in addressing issues that affect them, or direct them to the pathways that are going to lead to resolution of problems or support for their child. Some forms of advocacy are directed at the legal aspects of developmental conditions and disabilities, and offer legal advice to parents and families in order to access support or provision to accommodate their needs, support to which they may be legally entitled. Allocation of funding discussed in the previous chapter is one area where advocacy support is most widely sought, usually to challenge the institutions that control fund allocations.

To close this chapter, I emphasize that services need to be developed with a whole-child perspective but also have a regard for the interacting relationships between the child, family, school and wider community. If the focus is on engaging them and promoting self-efficacy as an essential route towards getting support and information about their child's needs, it is empowering them. Referring to an earlier quote 'when the need to do something is overwhelming', such involvement can only be positive.

Signposting activities for this chapter will take you to appropriate charities and local or regional organizations where specific parent advice can be located.

In Chapter 9, I give context to the emerging structures that are demanded by the Children and Families Bill (2013) and give some clarification to the development of the EHCP, while bringing together many of the issues discussed throughout these chapters.

Signposts to parent advocacy and support

The National Parent Partnership Network: www.parentpartnership.org.uk (accessed 2 July 2013).

IPSEA: www.IPSEA.org.uk (accessed 29 July 2013).

Council for Disabled Children: www.councilfordisabledchildren.org.uk (accessed 20 July 2013).

Every Disabled Child Matters (EDCM) in partnership with the Children's Trust: www.edcm.org.uk (accessed 2 January 2014).

For fathers, information can be found at: www.fatherhoodinstitute.org (accessed 19 July 2013).

Summary

- Changes in practice can be achieved at a low cost through a changed model of shared responsibilities and professional partnerships in the delivery of support and services. Local service providers should look to 'pool budgets' and work across agencies to identify and meet needs early.
- Working across agencies, developing professional communities, working with *both* parents where possible, developing policy underpinned by social learning rationale, in that we learn from others in different ways, can make a lasting impact on *all* parties involved.
- Recognize that families who are coping with a special need or disability have to see an attractive currency for engaging in professional/parent partnerships, enabling the development of self-advocacy and confidence in their self-efficacy skills.

- Be aware of parent vulnerability where behavioural responses to specific learning difficulties in the child may, over time, result in impairments in family structures and family functioning around the child, and cause a complex disturbance in the dynamics of the family.
- Know that some remedies, treatments and intervention programmes may not be in the best interests of the child or family, may be costly and have little evidence attached that shows positive efficacy as a result of their application. Professionals need to know how to discriminate between the empirically tested and the anecdotally 'sponsored' 'fads or miracle cures'.
- Know that professionals should strive to develop parents' self-efficacy and self-advocacy skills and support them in their own efforts to seek help and support for their children's needs.
- Understand that where parents lack confidence, encouraging their membership in wider advocacy groups to use collective pressure and guidance can lead to them accessing entitlements and rights to support for their child or children.

Chapter 9   The way forward: promoting integrative practice

> **Intended learning outcomes**
>
> At the end of this chapter you will
>
> * understand the concept of joint commissioning;
> * have a knowledge of the legislated 'duty' requirement for local authorities and health, education, health and social care services to ensure and promote integrated practices;
> * understand the responsibilities of the 'Local Offer'; have a knowledge of local services available for children and young people with SEN, and including those who are disabled;
> * understand the importance of Part three of the Children and Families Bill 2013–2014 which decribes statutory rights and protections for the child and for parents;
> * be aware of legislation that acts to support vulnerable children such as children with a developmental disorder as described in this book;
> * understand the single system of support from birth to 25 for all children and young people with SEN and their families;
> * be aware of the processes involved in the preparation of an EHCP for the child or young person with an EHCP; and
> * understand how a positive working model can, through a multi-professional team and collaboration across school and health services, effect beneficial outcomes for the child and the professionals involved.

Introduction

In this chapter I begin by outlining major reforms to the 2013–2014 Children and Families Bill, integrated service provision for vulnerable children with SEN. Local authority functions that aim to ensure rights and support for children with disabilities are described. The making of an EHCP, its legislative function and multi-professional service management of the plan is then described. Matters arising from the 2012 Health and Social Care Act are briefly summarized and reforms contextualized within the ecological systems model. Together legislation has brought management of health, well-being, social care and special or additional educational needs firmly into the local arena where the potential for partnerships and pooled resources will shape service provision.

Statutory responsibility alone though cannot produce a positive professional model of frontline 'local' services. Rapidly changing conditions, new legislation, new patterns of working and different consumer expectations will present a challenge. I conclude then by bringing together points made throughout these chapters, to look at building collaboration through consensus, to cross local government, education and the NHS boundaries and forge new partnerships. A skill-mix framework to support the client, the child or young person, affected by an adverse developmental trajectory or a disability, is proposed; and places the individual at the centre of evolving dynamic systems. I close by highlighting the established assets and positive qualities embedded in the universal health visiting service that could provide the impetus to change by crossing boundaries, sharing practice, costs and expertise with a range of across-professional practitioners.

Changing the system

The focus throughout this guide has been children and young people with developmental anomalies, and diagnostic and support systems around these children and their families. I started out in Chapter 1 by looking at the dynamics of the universal health service in England and the UK, and marked out through an ecological systems model, the progression towards community-based and integrated service models of support. At the national macro level, policy change that put the child at the heart of health care and delivery of support has evolved. The Children Act (2004) provided the legislative foundation and shifted political and organizational influences to the most recent model where needs and support for those with additional needs are to be met by local service providers.

In England, health, care and education services also have a legislated edict to promote integrated services locally. Local authorities and other policy makers within systems are required to make a step change in how they approach, and join up, early assessment and identification of developmental anomalies, often the first indicator of an adverse developmental trajectory.

At the macro level, the legal restructuring can transform what has to happen, through a single system for assessment, a framework I summarize here, along with the prescribed function and maintenance of the EHCP.

Legislative restructuring

The Children and Families Bill replaces Part IV of the 1996 Education Act that is concerned with children with SEN. This becomes law when the Bill is passed following Royal Assent in 2014. It then becomes the Children and Families Act 2014.

This legislation:

- replaces the 'statementing' system described in Chapter 1, with Education, Health and Care plans;
- extends statutory rights and protection for the child beyond school from 0–25 years;
- allows for support provision for the individual to be maintained in adulthood;
- strengthens the duties to cooperate across health, education and care agencies; and
- demands jointly commissioned cross-locality services.

Part three of the Bill is concerned with SEN reforms to statutory rights and protection, and aims to:

- raise aspirations;
- put children, young people and parents at the centre of decisions;
- extend greater choice and control over *what* sort of support; and
- give families and young people the offer of a personal budget and financial resources through which to manage their child's needs.

Crucially here though, is the requirement for LAs and health services to commission education, health and social care services jointly and a requirement to:

- support and involve parents, children and young people in the assessment process, making, reviewing and developing of an EHCP;
- agree what advice and information is to be provided about education, health and care provision, by whom, to whom and how much advice is to be provided (TSO 2013);
- get LAs to publish a clear and transparent 'local offer' of services to support children and young people with SEN and their families;
- encourage greater cooperation between LAs and a range of partners including schools, academies, colleges, other LAs and services with a remit to provide health and social care; and
- promote mediation to resolve disagreements through a single point of appeal.

The legislative changes extend to England and Wales but only have effect in respect of children and young people *from* England, and apply to the English education, health and social care agencies. Welsh agencies have duties under this legislation, only in respect of providing support for children and young people from England, but who are being educated in schools in Wales.

These reforms then emphasize the central role of the NHS, place stronger duties to promote health and well-being of children who have SEN, demand the delivery of joined-up integrated health and social care, and demand the provision of services identified in EHCPs including education provision (ibid.: 43–47). In Clause 42(4) the legal duty on health commissioners to arrange the health services that an LA specifies in the EHCP is outlined. If health services fail to arrange these services then parents or young people can legally challenge them in the law courts.

Partnerships also include a greater link to voluntary charities and community organizations contracted by the DfE to provide services concerning SEN and disability. These include the Council for Disabled Children (CDC) and organizations representing a range of disabilities and disorders including autism, dyslexia, sensory and multi-sensory impairment, low-incidence complex needs, SLCN, as well as many charities and advocacy organizations.

The local offer

The local offer for children and young people with SEN sets out the support that is available in an area for children and young people who have SEN. There is a legal demand for transparency with all local authorities required to publish, review and revise regularly their provision for those with a SEN and an EHC. Additionally though the local offer has to also publish support available for children and young people with SEN who do *not* have an EHCP. Included information in the 'local offer' is what health and social care provision can be expected from schools and colleges from their delegated budgets. Local authorities and clinical commissioning groups also have to make arrangements for commissioning services for children and young people with SEN whether they have an EHCP or not. Each authority also must publish regularly comments received from children and young people about the provision in the local offer and an LA in England may request the cooperation of any of the following bodies:

- another LA;
- a youth offending team;
- the NHS Commissioning Board;
- a clinical commissioning group;
- a Local Health Board;
- an NHS Trust or NHS Foundation.

The (0–25) Special Educational Needs Code of Practice 2013 offers guidance for meeting the needs of children with a SEN and a framework to inform professionals how the legal framework operates (Children and Families Bill 2013: Section 66 and 67). It describes the single category of need that replaced 'School Action' and 'School Action Plus'. It is also stressed here that it is a guidance document to which all parties concerned must have a regard, including:

- local authorities in England;
- the governing bodies of schools;
- the governing bodies of institutions within the further education sector;
- the proprietors of academies;
- the management committees of pupil referral units;
- the proprietors of institutions approved by the Secretary of State under section 41 (independent special schools and special post-16 institutions: approval);
- providers of relevant early years education;

- the NHS Commissioning Board;
- clinical commissioning groups;
- NHS Trusts;
- NHS foundation trusts; and
- Local Health Boards.

This code may also be revised from time to time and every current version of the code must be published.

The 2012 Health and Social Care Act brought about many changes including:

- the abolition of Primary Care Trusts and Strategic Health Authorities;
- GPs given the responsibility for commissioning via Clinical Commissioning Groups;
- LA to establish Health and Wellbeing boards as a part of the framework for cooperation between councils and health agencies;
- local *Healthwatch* independent organizations established April 2013 to facilitate patient involvement in quality control and local planning, giving patients a regional voice;
- *Healthwatch* England established – a national body to overview quality control and present collective views of people about the NHS and social care services to influence national policy, advice and guidance;
- Health and Wellbeing Boards given responsibility to carry out strategic needs, assessments and then produce a Joint Health and Wellbeing strategy based on this assessment, stipulating how they will meet the needs identified;
- provision to carry a duty to develop integrated working practices;
- expanded NICE functions; and
- the establishment of the Health and Social Care Information Centre.

The Education Healthcare Plan (EHCP)

Under this legislation, where a child has (or probably has) SEN, the duty of health authorities to bring him/her to the attention of the LA is laid out (ibid.: Part 3); and functionally 'a clinical commissioning group, NHS trust or NHS foundation trust' must address his/her needs. An LA in England must exercise its functions to provide integrated services and arrangements about the education, health and care provision for children and young people who have SEN. Where an LA is preparing an EHCP for the child or young person it must ensure that it provides for the individual concerned to be educated in a maintained nursery school, mainstream school or post-16 institution unless that is incompatible with

- the wishes of the child's parent or the young person; or
- the provision of efficient education for others.

(ibid.: Part 3 (33) (1) (2))

Conditions and duties are also laid out for children and young people with SEN but no EHCP (ibid.: 34: (1) to (10)). In England, an assessment of EHC needs can be requested from the LA by the child's parents, the young person or a person acting on behalf of a school or post-16 institution. The EHCP has to be maintained for the post-16 transition period (16–19) and cover further education, apprenticeships and training support (19–25). An EHC needs assessment is an assessment of the educational, health and social care needs of a child or young person, and when a request is made to an LA the authority must, after consultation with the parent, determine whether it may be necessary for special educational provision to be made for the individual in accordance with an EHCP. Regulations governing this process are clearly laid down (ibid.: Part 3 (36) lines 19–39). Where, following assessment, it is deemed necessary for special educational provision to be made in accordance with an EHCP, this has to be prepared and maintained. An EHCP is a plan specifying:

- the child's or young person's SEN;
- the outcomes sought for him or her;
- the special educational provision required by him or her;
- any health care and social care provision reasonably required by the learning difficulties and disabilities, which result in him or her having SEN.

It may also specify other health and social care provision reasonably required by the individual, and base all decisions with a regard to his or her age. Regulation of how the plan is to be prepared in draft form, by whom it should viewed, be a party to its adoption and the duration of its maintenance are clearly stipulated in the Bill (ibid.: Part 3 Sections 38–47). Personal budgets, discussed earlier in Chapter 7, are to be prepared by the LA, with a view to the child's parent or the young person being involved in securing provision of support needs stipulated in the EHCP. Section 48 of the Bill outlines how this provision is organized, what it can access and how resources are allocated/services are paid for.

Provision must be made through *Joint Commissioning Arrangements*. Education, health and care provision means:

- special educational provision;
- health care provision; and
- social care provision.

Joint commissioning arrangements must include arrangements for considering and agreeing the EHC provision that is reasonably required by the learning difficulties and disabilities which result in the children and young people having a SEN, as well as what education, health and care provision is to be made, by whom and how much. Also, the routes to resolve complaints; procedures for ensuring the settlement of disputes between all parties concerned; and a time limit for such complaints has to be published.

This legislation brings together the demands and duties of earlier reforms (Local Government and Public Involvement in Health Act 2007) whereby LAs have a duty regarding the assessment of relevant needs and joint health and well-being strategy. This consolidates the due process, and partnership, for delivering special EHC provision of services or facilities for any children and young people who have SEN. LAs also have a duty to review any provision, must consult children and young people and their parents and, if in school, the governing bodies, proprietors of any academy involved plus any other agency involved in each specific case. Partnership cooperation is emphasized throughout the Children and Families Bill.

Appeals, mediation and dispute resolution

These can be dealt with first through the First-tier Tribunal appeal mechanism that gives the child's parents or young person the right to appeal against a decision *not* to secure an EHC needs assessment. A due process has to be followed (ibid.: Section 50: 1–6) and mediation mechanisms (ibid.: Section 51: 1–8) are laid out to facilitate this. An authorized mediation adviser in this case is an independent person who can provide information and advice about pursuing mediation with an LA, and it should be stressed that a person who is employed by an LA in England is *not* independent. Local authorities also have a duty to give due process for resolving disagreements (ibid.: Section 52: 1–9). For the first time, the Secretary of State has advocated a pilot for enabling children in England to:

- appeal to the First-tier Tribunal under section 50;
- make a claim to the First-tier Tribunal under Schedule 17 to the Equality Act 2010 (disabled children enforcement) that a responsible body in England has contravened Chapter 1 of Part 6 of that Act because of the child's disability.

(ibid.: 53: lines 10–14)

In the event of this becoming the case, it would indeed put the young people at the very heart of their care and support delivery and provision to meet their additional needs.

I propose here key features that could augment multi-agency and community support, and could facilitate participation, not exclusion, of the children with a developmental disorder or disability. Underpinning concepts I propose as fundamental in planning such a model are reciprocity (Bronfenbrenner 1979) and 'socialness' or social capital (Putnam 2000: 19), both of which can foster engagement across, and within, systems. First discussed in Chapter 7 I reiterate that social capital encapsulates belonging to, and existing within, the relational bonds of society and its social networks. Social or community members then are essentially 'stakeholders' in their society where these relational bonds between individuals, families and groups in the community are strong. Professionals need not only be engaged socially themselves, but also promote and foster social engagement in clients; the case study presented in the previous chapter presents examples of how this can be achieved. If clients do *not* engage in social enterprise or community, they remain 'the problem' and limit the extent to which they become involved in solutions.

Health and education is where multi-professional planning should begin and with children in all early years settings, when features of a developmental anomaly are first becoming apparent. Promoting, planning, delivering, monitoring and evaluating cross-agency support needs to be shared and stringent, and *the social and emotional well-being for children and young people* pathway (NICE Pathways 2012) offers another route through which to build a strategy, policy or framework for the commissioning of services. Specialists in health can contribute broadly to education policy and practices. The TAC described in Chapter 6 provides one such initiative that has, and can, make a positive contribution in this area. A team can be enlarged and become a team around the family (TAF) or team around the school (TAS) where all the children with additional needs in a school are helped. Current policy deviates only marginally from these models, with 'in progress' guidance offered through the

Children and Families Bill (2013–2014) and the revised (0–25) Special Educational Needs Code of Practice 2013 referenced above.

In terms of promoting health and well-being, education and health should be inextricably linked, as the whole school approach to dealing with social and emotional health and well-being has shown. The Social and Emotional Aspects of Learning programme (SEAL) (DfES 2007: 5–6) has produced many different models of delivery, and has successfully embraced school nurses, psychotherapists, psychologists and other across-team partners.

The rationale underpinning the SEAL programme is that it promotes development in five domains proposed by Goleman's (1995) model of emotional intelligence. These are:

- self-awareness – knowing and valuing the self;
- self-regulation – how to manage and express emotions; how to cope with change;
- motivation – working towards goals, promoting resilience and optimism;
- empathy – understanding the thoughts and feelings of others; and
- social skills – building and maintaining relationships; solving problems.

Reflecting on the features of developmental disorders presented earlier, the value of such a programme to children with social skills or social communication problems, or those experiencing problems associated with specific developmental disorders, should become obvious.

Such a programme allows for the development of emotional literacy that gives the young person the language through which to clearly communicate feelings and emotion. It thus enables individuals to express more coherently the difficulties they are experiencing and the impact on their psychosocial functioning. The programme can underpin individual or small group intervention programmes, while also being appropriate for furthering the development of a commitment to whole school ethos of care and community, and that nurtures within its framework the concepts of socialness and reciprocity. A SEAL culture can be developed, across teams and services, can form the basis of continuing professional development (CPD) and is particularly pertinent where health, social care and educators have shared goals and responsibilities, want to develop integrated practices and work in partnership across a range of professionals. It would also facilitate a multi-agency package, delivered in a range of settings, to support greater inclusion of children with additional needs and lead to better outcomes for vulnerable groups per se.

As seen in Chapter 6, children with a developmental disorder or disability are vulnerable at certain times in their lives, at the early years stage and under the age of five years. All those included in the joint commissioning services in an LA should be part of the action taken. This includes:

- clinical commissioning groups;
- health and well-being boards;
- NHS Commissioning Board (until 2015); and
- public health, children's services, education and social services within local authorities.

Leadership commitment to developing joint policies and procedures and promoting the use of a school-health-community charter could aid professionals committed to working jointly towards:

- engaging health and education officials, teachers, pupils, parents and community leaders in an effort to develop inclusive practices for all regardless of a developmental disorder or disability;
- providing a safe environment that promotes healthy, inclusive physical and psychosocial well-being for all children; involving CAMHS in a *proactive* role not *reactive*;
- providing effective health education across the community wherein the child or young person is placed;
- providing access to a range of health services, and working with educators to ensure continuity across provision and situation can be achieved;
- implementing joint policies and practices across health, education and care;
- valuing the parents' role as 'expert' in understanding and managing their child's needs and difficulties; and capitalizing on this to educate those who 'care for' and support the child or young person; and
- engaging the community with charities representing recognized support advocacy groups and specific disabilities (e.g. NAS, ADHD/ADDISS).

Changing the practice

Educating teachers and paraprofessionals in the delivery of rudimentary, but vital, intervention could work, particularly where trained specialists, such as SLTs, are a scarce resource. By providing members of a school community with the tools they need could provide an alternative modus operandi that would benefit those children with a need. While acknowledging that language delay and language disorders do present a need for early identification by well-qualified specialists, there is also a need for early, regular and consistent intervention exercises that could be delivered by a trained paraprofessional.

Attention and behavioural difficulties, too, impact on, and impede, learning for the child with learning difficulties and class peers that can often produce negative long-term outcomes for the child through permanent exclusion from school. Managing arising 'in-school' difficulties could be the focus of a collaboration programme around the child, between psychological services, CAMHS, health professionals and those professionals who manage behaviour in schools.

Identifying 'at-risk' children in schools must also be a shared responsibility, as some of the learning difficulties described may only manifest when the demand for specific social situations changes, or when cognitive processes are required for specific skill acquisition (e.g. reading). To reiterate, idiosyncratic strategies mastered by the child or young person are often well developed in order to disguise learning difficulties, and these will without doubt eventually 'let them down'. Often teacher observations will also confirm a parent's 'gut feelings' but to recognize specific problems, teachers too need to be aware of what to look for. The parent, family and the health professionals need to share information about the child, and it is important too that teachers should receive training about specific congenital disorders.

Providing in-service awareness training for teachers about specific developmental disorders would not only aid early recognition of difficulties but could also alert them to potential impediments to learning that a child may present with. HVs or school nurses too could undertake a school audit, to assess areas of need and glean information about where additional training could be offered for teachers. Through this, whole school responsibility and strategies can be developed through which difficulties that can arise in the school environment can be circumvented.

A school audit could identify where areas of emotional and behavioural well-being need to be addressed and promoted through health education programmes. Bullying, violence or aggression are also elements in which a school can be experiencing problems that may, or may not, involve pupils with specific disorders or disabilities. Dealing with these too could be a shared responsibility between health, CAMHS professionals, teachers and paraprofessionals such as teaching assistants and school counsellors. Disorders such as ADHD are reported as being under-diagnosed in the UK. In this domain there is a need for primary and secondary care services to work efficiently together to manage core symptoms of ADHD. With reported delays of between nine months and five years, from families first voicing concerns and an ADHD diagnosis being given by a specialist (Klasen and Goodman 2000), the crucial key to improving such a situation would appear to be improved awareness and education.

Policies and procedures should be planned in unison with a range of service providers and policy should always reflect practice. They must also be developed so that the 'whole child' must also have a regard for the interacting relationships between the child, family and community. Explicit pro-social values need to be encouraged and demonstrated with the families of children with a disorder or disability. Self-help advocated in the previous chapter can be taught with guided support, and families have shown they can effectively engage in the management of their child's needs, which the personal budget or direct payment scheme demands.

Identifying the strengths of the family as well as the risks, and developing their 'social capital' or what they can bring to forge a positive involvement with the wider community, can improve and integrate the family's relationship with structures in society. It cannot be overstated that those who live with, and cope with, the daily demands of a child with a disorder or disability really are 'experts' in the needs of that child. Members of the family should be encouraged and directed towards sharing that experience with others. Joining or starting a support group, contributing towards a school health and pastoral project or talking to other parents recently faced with the same diagnosis they were once faced with are just a few ways in which parents are on the way to being a part of the solution and not just the problem.

In conclusion, in the first instance, issues around developmental disorders should be addressed by:

- raising awareness of such disorders through the training of those involved with infants and toddlers; e.g. HV, FNP, adults involved in early years childcare;
- helping parents to recognize anomalies in their child's developmental progress;
- educating the family GP and Practice or Health Centre Nurses about developmental disorders; and
- a multi-agency approach to working with parents to develop positive self-advocacy and self-efficacy skills – remove the dependency on one service to resolve problems.

The EHCP development and responsibilities are moving service providers forwards and, fundamentally, place the NHS in a pivotal role, but with the explicit message being that shared responsibilities *must* underpin service provision. Greater freedom has been given to local providers to move away from 'top-down' local dictates. Rather, change should be implemented, instead, through 'bottom-up', service-led provision, to meet additional needs of this group of vulnerable children and young people.

Change needs more than legislation. Local policies need to be developed, particularly with this vulnerable group in mind, that have a regard for the impact on their families; consider how they will be affected by policies; look at the ways in which families contribute to the issues; and, most important, consider how families can be involved in solutions. Taking a family impact perspective is not the same as family policy, where policy is designed to have specific effects on the family. Instead, it seeks to identify, and take account of, implicit and unintended consequences that policies have on families (Cadigan and Alberts 2009).

Evaluation of practice should strive to look beneath the surface, to identify not only intended but also unintended outcomes of policy. Frontline service professionals need to develop reflective practices, to examine their own value systems in any evaluation of outcomes derived from policy and professional practice. Here, social modelling can provide an instrument though which to apply scrutiny. The ecological model I described at the outset allows for recognition of the effect of interactions in overlapping contexts across each system in which the child and its family members are directly involved. It also takes account of neighbourhood and settings such as childcare and school, as well as systemic influences from direct interaction or influence from society, culture and social policy. These can be seen to have a significant effect on the individual, the family unit and the local community; through reciprocal bidirectional interactions and influences, change operates both ways.

Through the concept of a chronosystem, it is possible to see that in systems within the public health service, there have been numerous initiatives over time, some alluded to in these chapters. Many have disappeared, but not all have been cut, archived or disbanded. An evolving 'different' service has emerged, and current or future good practice must take account of what has gone before. Even as the concluding pages of this book are being written, so too are new policies and initiatives. Laws will become amended, and the outcome from case law will also impact on further and continuing change. Flexibility and diversity are two guiding principles in good practice, and established fundamental qualities of the HV service.

For the HV service the expansion programme outlined in Chapter 1 will, it is claimed, result in the HV 'having the time to provide parents with critical health and development advice' (Health Visitor Implementation Plan Quarterly Progress Report July–September 2012: 3). A bold vision and laudable outcome that the HV workforce will look forward to I'm sure. Academic programmes however are committed to training HV professionals to a high standard, and to ensure a fit-for-purpose service. Other initiatives and strategic plans have been politically repackaged (e.g. HCP evolving as 'Giving all children a healthy start in life' available at www.gov.uk/government/policies/giving-all-children-a-healthy-start-in-life (DH 2013)); and call on the HV service to provide additional support and intervention to those families who require them.

Intended to deliver the biggest reforms for children and young people with SEN and/or disabilities since the 1981 Education Act, a central aim of legislative reforms is to address disadvantages faced by vulnerable children and young people by transforming special education, health and social care (Children and Families Bill 2013). There is an enforced duty from the government of the day for cooperation and joint commissioning of education, health and social care within a single assessment of the child. To this end, a reciprocal duty of joint commissioning between education and health and the evolving collaboration that was introduced in Chapter 1 has reached summation.

In the Children and Families Bill (2013) improving choice for young people with SEN and their parents is made explicit through a clause that requires local authorities to prepare a 'personal budget' (ibid.: Section 48: 1–5) for children or young people with an EHCP. How the personal budget or direct payments will operate in practice is little understood and pilot programmes, still developing approaches to implement the scheme, do not report back to the Coalition Government until the end of September 2014.

Conclusion

- To understand and assist the individual and their family, the influences across all contexts, systems and environments must be recognized.
- The child or young person with a developmental disorder and his/her family will have an influence on systems *outside* of themselves.
- As the child develops, the individual interacts more directly with more systems.
- The macro systems (e.g. society and policies within) may not interact directly with the child and the family, but they still hold a significant influence. The EHCP and the Children and Families Bill (2013) are a pertinent example of the extent of these influences.
- The most effective approach to early identification and appropriate intervention for the child with a developmental disorder and/or disability and the family is one where a combination of professional inputs operates across all systems or levels.

We have seen that limitations and forces within systems can act for, and against, the best interests of the child and family concerned here, and decisions have to be reconciled by professionals. The bidirectional influences in systems show us how, through no fault of their own, professionals have to deliver frontline services and administer support across several systems. They have to justify to others decisions made by others that may be in total conflict with their own professional views, and may even act against the best interest of the child and the family.

Decisions about allocation of resources, as the review of funding models in Chapter 7 showed, can be based on arbitrary criteria (e.g. free school meals). Allegedly, institutions worldwide have also been found to be over-claiming funds, in practices described as 'fiscal' or 'perverse incentives'. In the UK in 2011, the Secretary of State for Education suggested schools had wrongly labelled thousands of children as requiring special educational teaching, and funding, when this really covered 'poor teaching and just naughty children' (*Daily Mail*, 9 March 2011) and 170,000 children were removed almost instantly from schools' SEN registers. Such is the vulnerability of socially constructed phenomenon. As illustrated in Chapter 3, this vulnerability impacts on socially described childhood disorders and classifications within diagnostic manuals. These as we have seen can be variable and dynamic. Definitions expand as our knowledge increases, but can also fluctuate according to events nationally and internationally, while being far removed from the immediate environs of the individual child or his or her family (e.g. AS 'disappearing' from the *DSM-5* in 2013).

Primary and secondary impacts need to be recognized as these 'impacts' go beyond just the child who has the disorder or disability. Family tensions that result impact on parents' relationships and siblings, and the longer-term issues that can arise, for all members of the family, place more than just the child 'at risk' of presenting with dysfunctional social and emotional behaviours.

The principle of guided self-help is what frontline service providers should be offering in supporting the parents and families of children with disabilities or complex developmental needs. In the move forward, support must be promoted, not assistance, and developing competences and resilience in young people and their parents has got to be a priority. How otherwise can children and young people become more independent, take greater control and exercise more choice over support to manage their specific needs?

Evidence presented throughout these chapters has shown how earlier models, guidance and codes of practice have also produced genuinely supportive initiatives. To utilize these features that represent good practice, when forming and reforming future models would, to my mind, make sense. In the planning of support for children and young people with additional needs, it is possible to have a regard for current governing legislation, without having to abandon former practices that have also been shown to be effective.

Clinical and specialist skills need to be reflective, and based on current evidence-based research that has never been so readily available. Internet access means information can be located almost instantly, but also needs to be filtered judiciously and claims made considered reflectively and cautiously. So too is the need to be informed about evolving legislation, initiatives and policies, all of which places yet more demands on the time of the frontline service providers and professionals.

Expanding services such as health visiting and school nurses alone is a start, but not enough. Changed practice within the systems, based on different ideologies, that produce a workforce that breaks down barriers and crosses professional boundaries, and that values *all* contributions, also needs to be adopted.

By including the strategies that are presented here, others have, by necessity, been excluded, but not disregarded. But the core understanding here is that those who are the frontline service providers have the skills, knowledge and motivation to do the best they can, for those with the greatest need. I hope this book has gone some way towards furthering that knowledge, and motivates the professional to seek out more for themselves.

Appendix

The Sally-Anne Test to investigate ToM

This test has been used in psychological research to investigate ToM. A ToM is the ability to understand your own and other people's beliefs, desires, intentions and emotions (see Chapter 5). In autism it has been proposed that lacking a ToM may explain some of the social and communication difficulties experienced by those with autism.

The test

- To start the test, two dolls, one called Sally and the other called Anne, are presented to the child.
- The child is then told Sally has a basket and Anne has a box.
- Next, the child is told that Sally puts a marble inside her basket and then Sally leaves and goes where she can no longer see her basket.
- While Sally is away Anne takes the marble from Sally's basket and puts it inside her box.
- The child is told that Sally comes back inside.
- To make sure the child understands the basics s/he is asked:

  Q1 Which one is Sally?
  Q2 Which one is Anne?
  Q3 Where is the marble now?
  Q4 Where was the marble in the beginning?

- Then comes the big question.
- The ToM question asks: Where will Sally look for her marble?
- If the child realizes that Sally will look for the marble in her own basket and not in the box, then the child can understand Sally's perspective and you can say the child has a ToM.

- If the child says that Sally will look for the marble in Anne's box then you could say the child does *not* have a ToM as the child does *not* appear to understand Sally's perspective and that Sally did *not* see Anne take the marble and put it inside the box. The results?

- The results below are from a frequently cited study (Baron-Cohen *et al.* 1985) that used the Sally Anne test with:

  a   children with autism;
  b   children with Down syndrome; and
  c   typically developing children.

- All of the children got the basic questions correct.

- In the ToM question, only four out of 20 children with autism got the question correct.

- Of the children with Down syndrome, 12 out of 14 got the question correct.

- Of the typically developing children, 23 out of 27 got the question correct.

- Over time results from studies showing that children with autism frequently get the ToM question incorrect offers a potential reason why they frequently present with social skills and communication difficulties.

Responses to self-answer activities

Activity 1.1: Internet and online search

The three main initiatives are:

- Wales: Welsh Assembly: Children and Young People: Rights to Action (2003);
- Scotland: Getting it Right for Every Child (GIRFEC) (2008); and
- Northern Ireland: Families Matter: Supporting Families in Northern Ireland (2007).

Activity 1.2: Developing reflective practices

a   This could be the ability to consider influential nature and nurture factors in the child's environment, child-rearing practices, the cultural context of the child and the family or the allocation of resources under 'local service agreements'. Who can access support and how?

b   i   *micro*system – HCP from 0–5 years: the biological factors in the family, parent(s), relationships between the family, the birth position of the child in the family; SS programme could be seen as replacing the extended family of more traditional child-rearing patterns.

   ii   *meso*system – monitoring and assessing child development through programmes as SGS II. Or the interrelationship between the parent and the immediate systems where the family are placed and function, e.g. HV, family practitioners, childcare workers.

   iii   *exo*system – events such as the UK economic recession, loss of employment, changes to benefits system, cuts in children's services, changed childcare arrangements, constraints of family budget, family tensions.

   iv   *macro*system – again the economic constraints affected policy and provision of services; cuts in expenditure, new political ethos effecting new policies.

   v   *chrono*system – the time frame through which to look at changes; was provision better/worse in the past or presently? How does today's provision compare to that of say 50 years ago? How are things going to change in the future?

c   The framework of this model of human development supports psychosocial and cultural enquiry to identify and examine social, political, economical, cultural, emotional and familial influences in the developmental environment. Thinking about two or three examples of child health issues that you have encountered, how useful would this model be to understand constraints, or opportunities, that affect change *for your client or their family*?

Activity 2.1: SAQs

a   Attachment is the earliest bond formed between children and their caregiver. An enduring emotional bond and connectedness.

b   Observation is the only practical way to study behaviour in small children.

c   In secure attachment the caregiver provides secure and dependable, consistent care. The infant is distressed when separated from the caregiver, but happy when she returns. In the infant with insecure attachment, s/he is not comfortable or confident that care will be reliable. It may be disorganized care, sporadic and the infant may seem apprehensive in the company of the caregiver.

d   Reciprocity is an interaction in a dyadic relationship between two people, e.g. the mother and the infant, where turn taking naturally occurs in an engagement situation. Cues are passed between them and responses build up into a non-verbal language that communicates the needs of the infant that are understood by the mother.

e   Naturalistic observation allows the researcher to observe a phenomenon in its natural environment, to look at behaviour, interactions and actions. One advantage is the setting, which may be familiar to the child being observed, and therefore comfortable. A disadvantage is that you cannot control the variables in the setting, variables that may be superfluous, distracting and/or limit the chance of replication in any other setting.

Activity 2.2: SAQs

a   The image of self is formed in response to information the young person perceives from within his or her setting/community/culture. The adolescent constantly appraises this feedback to shape how they perceive themselves against others. The rate of physical development, body changes, shape, height, size are all constantly weighed against 'norms' seen in peers and portrayed through the media.

b   A society's view of disability or difference: whether it follows a medical 'within child' blame model or 'social model' where impediments are removed in the environment to allow the identity of self to emerge in a positive way.

c   The ecological systems approach can reveal influences that are present in the nurturing environment, from the micro level and through systems up to, and included in, the *macro*system. These influences can impact at an unconscious level, and identify factors present in systems that affect the adolescent but where he or she is not present.

d   Three influences that shape self-identity are the family, peers and the cultural developmental context.

e   Ego-identity in Erikson's (1980/1994) model of psychosocial development refers to the conscious sense of self that we develop through social interaction. Ego-synthesis is achieved when the growing child becomes aware of his or her own way of mastering experience.

Activity 2.3: SAQs

a   A neuron is a nerve cell. The brain is made up of approximately 100 billion neurons. They contain cytoplasm, mitochondria and other 'organelles'. Neurons are similar to other cells in the body in as much as they are surrounded by a membrane and have a nucleus that contains genes.

b   Neuroscientists study at different levels at the:
   - Behavioural level: the neural basis of behaviour, what causes people and animals to do the things they do.
   - System level: the various parts of the nervous system such as the visual or auditory system. This could also include investigations of what parts of the brain are connected to other parts.
   - Local circuit level: the function of groups of neurons (nerve cells).
   - Single neuron level: what individual neurons do in relation to some 'event'. Also, what is contained within a single neuron or neurotransmitter studies.
   - Synapse level: what happens at the synapse.
   - Membrane level: what happens at ion channels on a neuronal membrane.
   - Genetic level: the genetic basis of neuronal function.

c   The three main parts of the brain are forebrain, midbrain and hindbrain.
   - The forebrain includes the several lobes of the cerebral cortex that control higher functions.
   - Midbrain functions include routing, selecting, mapping and cataloguing information, including information perceived from the environment and information that is remembered and processed throughout the cerebral cortex.
   - Hindbrain (rhombencephalon) in vertebrates is a developmental categorization of portions of the CNS.

d   Broca's area is located in the frontal part of the left hemisphere of the brain. One of the main areas of the cerebral cortex it contains motor neurons involved in the control of speech. It is also a section of the human brain that is involved in language processing, speech or sign production, and comprehension.

e   Growing and developing through use, myelination is use-dependent in the neurological process. Myelin is a fatty covering that grows along the axon and conducts synaptic activity. Acting as an insulator, it helps to increase the speed of synaptic activity, making fast and more efficient neurological activity.

f   The limbic system is a set of structures that form the border of the cortex, known also as the hindbrain. This set of structures support functions that include emotion, behaviour and long-term memory.

g   Wernicke's area is part of the cerebrum on the posterior section of the superior temporal gyrus, located in the left hemisphere; its specialized function is in the domain of language skills, comprehension or understanding.

h   The thick band of fibres that separate the cerebral hemispheres is the Corpus Callosum.

i   The motor cortex is located in the frontal lobe of the brain.

j   One theory about the phase of development often termed the 'terrible twos' is referred to as 'pruning': a selective process for selecting strong synapses that will become skill competencies in the child.

Another explanation draws from psychosocial and linguistic theories. In language and comprehension development, Wericke and Broca's areas do not develop simultaneously. Vygotsky's theory of thought and language also posits a 'gap' between language acquisition and cognitive thought that demands language. This 'gap' then can lead to frustration in the toddler who can know words, but does not fully comprehend what is being said to him/her, as s/he lacks the language to understand concepts.

Activity 3.1: Internet and online search

Different facets or types of memory or classifications of human memory and their functions can include

a   Short-term memory or 'working memory' is the capacity for holding a small amount of information in the mind so it is readily available but only for a very short period of time.

b   Working memory is the ability we have to hold in our mind, and mentally manipulate, information over very short periods of time – 'a mental workspace' (Gathercole *et al.* 2006).

c   Auditory memory is the ability to process information presented orally or received aurally, analyse it in the mind and store it to be recalled later. Important when developing mastery in language and literacy skills and/or following instructions.

d   Visual memory has a basic function to recall an object or visually sensed image once it has been removed from sight and, in literacy, it is recalling and recognizing words, or letters in words, accurately enough to understand the meaning each letter or word conveys.

e   Episodic memory (Tulving 1983) refers to the capacity to consciously remember experienced events and situations over the individual's developing life cycle. Helps us to recall places we have been to and things we have seen. It allows for mental travel back into the past and cognitively think about the future.

f   Semantic memory (Tulving 1983) allows us to store more specific memories and/or general knowledge.

g   Long-term memory stores vast amounts of information and holds over much longer periods of time than it does in the short-term memory.

h   Procedural memory is the memory of a sequence of events that are essential to perform a task, and that we can recall *unconsciously*, for example, driving a car, riding a bicycle, making a cup of tea, etc.

i   Declarative memory is the memory of facts and events that can be *consciously* recalled. It is the explicit memory because it consists of information that we explicitly store and retrieve. It can be subdivided into *episodic memory* and *semantic memory.*

j   Sensory memory allows us to retain impressions of sensory information long after the original stimulus is withdrawn. It acts as a buffer for sensory information received through sight, touch, smell, taste and hearing. If a stimuli is perceived, it becomes stored, such as the smell of a particular perfume or an unpleasant smell such as vomit, and when the smell is re-presented at another time, it can consciously stimulate quite accurate recall of the original stimuli, the event, surroundings and circumstances where it occurred.

k   Spatial memory is the memory subset responsible for storing and giving information about the individual's spatial orientation, where one is at any given moment in time, standing, sitting, walking, etc. It accumulates information from sensors, or proprioceptors, that send received signals through the skin and muscles to the brain, and informs where limbs are in respect to the space around them. At another level spatial memory can recall features, facts and directions in and around our environment through recalling features and landmarks from a previous visit.

l   The multi-component model of working memory (Baddeley and Hitch 1974). This model proposes working memory has three components: the *central executive*, the *phonological loop* and the *visuo-spatial sketchpad*. The central executive is responsible for the control and regulation of cognitive processes, binding and coordinating information from a number of sources; the phonological loop, sometimes referred to as the articulatory loop, deals with sounds or phonological information. This 'loop' has two parts, a short-term store for auditory memory traces that are subject to rapid decay, and an articulatory loop that can retrieve the memory trace. The visuo-spatial sketchpad holds information about what we see. It stores it temporarily and manipulates spatial and visual information aiding memory of objects such as shapes' patterns and colours. It is principally represented within the right hemisphere of the brain.

A simplified example of how this model works could be when receiving a phone call. The central executive, or powerhouse, brings together the task of answering the phone or responding to the stimuli presented (ringing tone). The caller asks you to phone them back and give you their number. By constantly repeating this to yourself you are activating the articulatory or phonological loop, in order to 'hold' the sound and the sequence of the numbers; you quickly find a pen and you make a visual representation by writing the numbers down. Writing it down involves using the visuo-sketchpad, plus a kinaesthetic or movement component. Recalling that number later you would use all components to remember, using the visuo-sketchpad with the executive function to coordinate all components of the task.

Activity 3.2: SAQs

a   Criticisms and/or weaknesses directed at a diagnostic manual could be:
   •   a congenital developmental disorder, often dependent on symptoms being 'matched' to criteria in a checklist/in a diagnostic manual, and/or when a particular skill area has not developed as expected;
   •   if a particular outcome is anticipated from the tests then it is possible to 'choose' the symptoms most indicative to a disorder;
   •   that manuals describe behaviour that ranges from normal to different from that of the normal achiever. Our understanding of 'normal' can vary very widely.
   •   categories of 'disorder' are socially defined and are dynamic. They change dependent *on the information of the time.*
   •   diagnostic procedures modify our expectations of what is, or is not, normal functioning and categories broaden over time.
b   The information both the *DSM-IV* or *ICD-10* give is a clear statement of what behaviours are observed in the child *at the time of an assessment*. It offers a good

starting point for an assessment, or a component of a wider assessment of difficulties, but a manual should *never* be the sole determinant of making a diagnosis.

c   The benefits of a manual are the shared consensuses about what sort of features or behaviours constitute specific developmental disorders. It also gives the prevalence of a condition or disorder; in populations of same-age children; in different cultures; and in developed countries such as the UK and Europe (*ICD-10/11*); or in the US and other nations (*DSM-IV/5*).

d   Physical developmental checks and psychometric tests, recommended for a child age six years with difficulties mastering spoken language, could include:
   • physical hearing and speech checks to establish that the child has no impediments to normal hearing, together with early SL history;
   • what is the child's home language?
   • did the child go through cooing and babbling, making sounds, attempting word sounds (e.g. 'dada'/'mama', 'bubba')?
   • a clinical check of the speech organs, swallowing, eating;
   • psychometric tests to check expressive language, best understood as the 'output' in language, and receptive language the 'input'. Expressive language skills or the use of sounds are words and sentences used to convey meaning to others or to communicate. Receptive language skills or the understanding of language can be in words and gestures. Both of these should be checked;
   • a profile of the child's strengths and weaknesses using a non-verbal cognitive processing investigation, e.g. Raven's Coloured Progressive Matrices (Raven 2003) would be useful.

e   Before using *any* test with a child under the age of ten years you should:
   • give the child the reason for a particular test;
   • access parental/guardian consent;
   • know who raised the concerns, why were they raised, and what the developmental concerns about the child are;
   • record any other noted milestone delays if any are absent; and
   • ask about birth history and family circumstances, birth position in the family, history of such difficulties in siblings/parents.

Activity 3.3: Reflective practice

There are numerous policies that point directly, and indirectly, to an expected professional standard of behaviour, and that lay down clear expectations from professionals delivering services and care to children and their families in a universal health service. The following represent *some* of them but there may be more depending on your particular practitioner role or field of expertise.

• NMC (2013) The Code: Standards of Conduct, Performance and Ethics for Nurses and Midwives. Downloaded from www.nmc-uk.org (accessed 20 July 2013).
• For HVs, the four principles of health visiting that underpin health visiting practice and policies. These can be found in Cowley, S. and M. Frost (2006). The Principles of Health Visiting: Opening the Doors to Public Health Practice in the 21st Century, London, CPHVA & UKSC.

Many of the standards and practice guide documents can be obtained from the NMC website www.nmc-uk.org/Publications/Standards (accessed 2 August 2013).

Other formal policies and standards of best practice include:

- local safeguarding policies;
- national safeguarding policies;
- lone worker policies;
- standards of proficiency for specialists, community public health nurses and HVs;
- medicine management standards;
- standards of proficiency for nurse prescribers (as some HVs are prescribers too);
- NMC standards;
- the Children's Plan;
- responsibilities, fitness to practice;
- healthy lives, brighter futures;
- equality and diversity strategies (NMC 2011, www.equalityhumanrights.com (accessed 23 June 2013)); and
- the Prep Handbook (NMC 2011).

Activity 5.1: SAQs

Features that may be identified in each – but to a lesser or greater degree are given below. Remember though no two children are the same even if they share the same diagnosis.

a   ASD/AS (1) (2) (3) (4) (7) (8) (9) (10) (11) (12) (13) (14) (15)
b   dyspraxia (1) (4) (5) (7) (8) (9) (10) (11)
c   dyslexia (1) (4) (5) (6) (8) (9) (10) (11) (12)
d   ADHD (1) (4) (5) (7) (8) (9) (10) (11)
e   RS (2) (3) (5) (6) (8) (9) (10) (11) (12) (14) (15) (16)
f   FASD (1) (4) (5) (8) (9) (10) (11) (12)
g   WBS (1) (4) (5) (7) (8) (9) (10) (11) (12) (13) (14) (15)

Activity 6.1: SAQs

Several aspects need to be looked at here. The legal situation, health needs, psychosocial and SEN.

a   For your professional advice: NICE Guidelines, referenced organizations in Chapter 4.2, the Directory and Appendix 2.
b   The mother could be referred to the family GP, a local support group or ADDISS; for legal guidance direct her to IPSEA or a supporting advocacy group. You could also recommend the NICE parent training programme www.nice.org.uk/cg72 (accessed 15 January 2014).
c   You should ask the boy where *he* would prefer to meet, e.g. at home/school/youth centre/health centre. To access his perspective allow him to lead the interview and tap into a point that he raises and from where you think you could begin to access deeper information.

d   Access more information from organiazations such as IPSEA. Contact the school; talk to his immediate teachers about ADHD; ensure the boy's legal entitlements are not being compromised.

e   Foster a school/health collaboration by developing a TAC; work with the school on some in-service training for the 'whole school'. Involve CAMHS nurse/school nurse. It is a whole school issue.

f   To form a multi-discipline response team to resolve this issue you could build support around the child and involve representatives from the school nurse service, the HV, the school's pastoral staff and senior leaders; the psychology service; or a representative from a charity support group.

Activity 7.1: Reflective practice

Barriers to good practice

- Resistance to change.
- A lack of knowledge or skills.
- Not respecting those from other professions.
- Holding prejudiced and narrow views.
- Being indiscreet.

Personal qualities

- Knowing how to listen to others, regardless of age.
- Able to show understanding.
- Able to empathize.
- Know when to ask for, or seek, help for yourself.
- An ability to work in a team.
- Able to listen to and respond to parental concerns.
- Be a good communicator.

Professional qualities

- An understanding of the tools and processes that support multi-agency, integrated working.
- Knowing and taking account of legislation and ethical issues inbved.
- Have an understanding of 'normal' developmental changes in children.
- An ability to work together effectively supporting colleagues.
- Keeping up to date with evidence-based research and knowledge.
- Able to consider the broader needs of the family and siblings.

Activity 8.1: Internet and online search

a   Refer to NICE guidelines http://guidance.nice.org.uk/CG128 Appendix C Signs and symptoms of possible autism: Table 1 in particular.

b   A good starting point would be to contact Independent Panel of Special Education Advice – IPSEA advice line at www.ipsea.org (accessed 2 January 2014).

c   There are several sources that may be useful, and will deal with questions the parent wants answering over time. Initially though for succinct information for families go to *Contact a family* available at www.cafamily.org.uk/medical-infor-mation/conditions/w/williams-syndrome (accessed 2 January 2014). Caution is advised initially about website information outside of the UK. The above site will give parent support group contact details, which can be invaluable in the first few weeks after a diagnosis. A further excellent source is the Williams Syndrome Foundation information available at www.williams-syndrome.org.uk (accessed 4 January 2014).

d   The parents need to be guided to the scientific evidence available that refutes the connection most strongly. You could start with NHS information available at www.nhs.uk/Conditions/vaccinations/Pages/mmr-vaccine.aspx (accessed 4 January 2014). For links to scientific research papers and findings the National Centre for Immunisation Research and Surveillance (NCIRS) site offers some clear and useful information available at www.ncirs.edu.au/immunisation/education/mmr-decision/faq-safety.php FAQ 2 MMR Decision Aid (accessed 23 December 2013).

e   First line of reference could be NICE CG72 Attention Deficit Hyperactivity Disorder (ADHD) available at www.nice.org.uk/cg72 (accessed 5 January 2014).

f   Guidance for parents can be found through IPSEA available at www.ipsea.org. Guidance about the 'Local Offer' and what support it offers the child with learning difficulties can be found on all local authority websites in England. NAS information is also available at www.autism.org.uk (accessed 2 January 2014).

g   The BDA offers a national helpline about dyslexia, details available at www.bdadyslexia.org.uk (accessed 2 January 2014). Evidence from clinical trials for ADHD treatment is also available at www.nhs.uk/Conditions/Attention-deficit-hyperactivity-disorder/Pages/clinical-trial.aspx (accessed 2 January 2014). A parent helpline is also offered at www.youngminds.org.uk (accessed 2 January 2014).

h   NHS *Choices* site offers 'first stop' information available at www.nhs.uk/conditions/leaky-gut-syndrome/Pages/Introduction.aspx (accessed 2 January 2014). The site also links to a review of the evidence undertaken in 2006.

i   The NICE information 'ADHD Methyphenidate, Atomoxetine and Dexamfetamine (review) TA 98 and TA13' is a good place to start, available at http://guidance.nice.org.uk/TA98 (accessed 2 January 2014).

Glossary

Adverse developmental trajectory   an unfavourable or unusual developmental pathway

Atypical   not typical, often referring to autism where development is said to be atypical

Cognition   thought processes, mental action of learning and understanding

Congenital   present from birth

Developmental   changes over time

Disorder   a condition that disturbs normal functioning in specific areas, skills or body function

Dissonance   emotional discomfort about holding conflicting views or emotions; mentally agitated

Familial   factors within the family

Ideation   to have an idea or thoughts about an action

Pervasive disorder   affecting all development, e.g. cognition, coordination

Reciprocity   at one level an interrelationship between two persons, at another level, interactions between the individual and his/her community

Social modelling   producing a plan through which to look at underpinning systems in a particular society or population

Somatic   referring to the body and bodily functioning

Statute   laws and decrees made by government

References

Ainsworth, M. D. S. and S. M. Bell (1969). 'Some contemporary patterns in the feeding situation'. In A. Ambrose (ed.) *Stimulation in Early Infancy*. London, Academic Press, pp. 133–170.

Ainsworth, M., M. Blehar, E. Waters and S. Wall (1978). *Patterns of Attachmment: A Psychological Study of the Strange Situation*. Mahwah, NJ, Lawrence Erlbaum.

Ambitious about autism (2011). *Shaping Children's Services Together*. Downloaded from www.ambitiousaboutautism.org.uk/lib/liDownload/249/ShapingServicesTogether_Final_Proof.pdf (accessed 7 January 2014).

Amir, R., I. B. Van den Veyver, M. Wan, C. Q. Tran, U. Francke and H. Y. Zoghbi (1999). 'Rett syndrome is caused by mutations in X-linked MECP2, encoding methyl-CpG-binding protein'. *Nature Genetics*, 23, 185–188.

Amminger, G. P., G. E. Berger, M. R. Schafer, C. Klier, M. H. Friedrich and M. Feucht (2007). 'Omega-3 fatty acids supplementation in children with autism: a double-blind randomized, placebo-controlled pilot study'. *Biological Psychiatry*, 61 (4), 551–513.

APA (1994). *Diagnostic and Statistical Manual of Mental Disorders, Fourth Edition DSM-IV*. Washington DC, American Psychiatric Association.

APA (2000). *Diagnostic and Statistical Manual of Mental Disorders, Fourth Edition DSM-IV-TR (Text Revision)*. Washington DC, American Psychiatric Association.

APA (2013). *Diagnostic and Statistical Manual of Mental Disorders, Fifth Edition DSM-5*. Washington DC, American Psychiatric Association.

Armstrong, T. (2011). *Neurodiversity: Discovering the Extraordinary Gifts of Autism, ADHD, Dyslexia and Other Brain Differences*. Philadelphia, Da Capo Press.

Ausubel, D. P. (2002). *Theory and Problems of Adolescent Development*. New York, iUniverse-Writers Club Press.

Auyeung, B., S. Baron-Cohen, E. Ashwin, R. Knickmeyer, K. Taylor and G. Hackett (2009). 'Fetal testosterone and autistic traits'. *British Journal of Psychology*, 100, 11–22.

Ayres, A. J. (1972a). *Sensory Integration and Learning Disorders*. Los Angeles, CA, Western Psychological Services.

Ayres, A. J. (1972b). 'Improving academic scores through sensory integration'. *Journal of Learning Disabilities*, 5, 339–343.

Baddeley, A. and G. Hitch (1974). 'Working memory'. In G. H. Bower (ed.) *The Psychology of Learning and Motivation: Advances in Research and Theory*. New York, Academic Press, pp. 47–89.

Baird, G., T. Charman, A. Cox, S. Baron-Cohen, J. Swettenham, S. Wheelwright and A. Drew (2001). 'Screening and surveillance for autism and pervasive developmental disorders'. *Archives of Disease in Childhood*, 84, 468–475.

Bandura, A. (1977). *Social Learning Theory*. New York, General Learning Press.

Bandura, A. (1982). 'Self-efficacy mechanism in human agency'. *American Psychologist*, 37 (2), 122–147.

Bandura, A. (1986). *Social Foundations of Thought and Action: A Social Cognitive Theory.* Englewood Cliffs, NJ, Prentice Hall.

Bandura, A. (1989/1992). 'Social cognition theory'. *Annals of Child Development, Vol 6, Six Theories of Child Development.* In R. Vasta (ed.) *Six Theories of Child Development: Revised Formulations and Current Issues.* London, Jessica Kingsley Publishers, pp. 1–60.

Bandura, A. (1993). 'Perceived self-efficacy in cognitive development and functioning'. *Educational Psychologist*, 28 (2), 117–148.

Bandura, A. (1994). 'Self-efficacy'. In V. S. Ramachaudran (ed.) *Encyclopedia of Human Behavior*. New York, Academic Press, Vol. 4, pp. 71–81. (Reprinted in H. Friedman (ed.) *Encyclopedia of Mental Health*. San Diego, CA, Academic Press, 1998).

Barker, P. (1990). *Clinical Interviews with Children and Adolescents*. New York, W. W. Norton & Company.

Barkley, R. A. (1997). 'Behavioural inhibition, sustained attention, and executive functions: constructing a unifying theory of ADHD'. *Psychological Bulletin*, 12 (1), 65–94.

Barkley, R. A. (2003). 'Issues in the diagnosis of attention-deficit/hyperactivity disorder'. *Brain and Development*, 25, 77–83.

Baron-Cohen, S. (2002). 'The extreme male brain theory of autism'. *Trends in Cognitive Sciences*, 6 (6), 248–254.

Baron-Cohen, S., A. M. Leslie and U. Frith (1985). 'Does the Autistic child have theory of mind?' *Cognition*, 21, 37–46.

Baron-Cohen, S., F. J. Scott, C. Allison, J. Williams, P. Bolton, F. E. Matthews and C. Brayn (2009). 'Prevalence of autism-spectrum conditions: UK school-based population study'. *British Journal of Psychiatry*, 194, 500–509.

BASW (2012). *The Code of Ethics for Social Work: Statement of Principles*. Birmingham, The Policy, Ethics and Human Rights Committee, British Association of Social Workers.

Bateman, B., J. O. Warner, E. Hutchinson, T. Dean, P. Rowlandson, C. Gant, J. Grundy, C. Fitzgerald and J. Stevenson (2004). 'The effects of a double blind, placebo controlled, artificial food colourings and benzoate preservative challenge on hyperactivity in a general population sample of preschool children'. *Archives of Diseases in Childhood*, 89 (6), 506–511.

Bateson, K., J. Delaney and R. Pybus (2008). 'Meeting expectations: the pilot evaluation of the Solihull Approach Parenting Group'. *Community Practitioner*, 81, 28–31.

Batten, A., C. Corbett, M. Rosenblatt, L. Withers and R. Yuille (2006). *Autism and Education: The Reality for Families Today*. The National Autistic Society. Download from www.autism.org.uk (accessed 19 July 2013).

Bauman, M. and T. Kemper (2005). 'Neuroanatomic observations of the brain in autism: a review for future directions.' *International Journal of Developmental Neuroscience*, 23, 183–187.

Bercow, J. (2008). The Bercow Report: A Review of Services for Children and Young People (0–19) with Speech, Language and Communication Needs. DCSF. Download from http://dera.ioe.ac.uk/8405/1/7771-dcsf-bercow.pdf (accessed 19 July 2013).

Bettelheim, B. (1967). *The Empty Fortress: Infantile Autism and the Birth of the Self*. New York, The Free Press.

Beuren, A. J., J. Apitz and D. Harmjanz (1962). 'Supravalvular aortic stenosis in association with mental retardation and a certain facial appearance'. *Circulation*, 27, 1235–1240.

Bion, W. R. (1959). 'Attacks on linking'. In E. Bott Spillius (ed.) *Melanie Klein Today: Developments in Theory and Practice. Volume 1: Mainly Theory*. London, Routledge.

Bishop, D. (2008). Treating Reading Disability without Reading: Evaluating Alternative Intervention Approaches. BDA International Dyslexia Conference, April. Harrogate, Yorkshire.

Blackburn, C. (2009). FASD Building Bridges with Understanding: The Acquisition of Practitioner Knowledge in Relation to the Management of Support of Children with Foetal

Alcohol Syndrome and Related Disorders. Downloaded from www.nofas-uk.org (accessed 31 December 2013).

Blackburn, C., B. Carpenter and J. Egerton (2009). *Facing the Challenge and Shaping the Future for Primary and Secondary Age Students with Foetal Alcohol Spectrum Disorders (FAS-eD Project)*. NOFAS-UK. Downloaded from www.nofas-uk.org (accessed 15 July 2013).

Blakemore, S. J. and S. Choudhury (2006). 'Development of the adolescent brain: implications for executive function and social cognition'. *Journal of Child Psychology and Psychiatry*, 47 (3), 296–312.

Bobb, A. J., F. X. Castellanos, A. M. Addington and J. L. Rapoport (2005). 'Molecular genetic studies of ADHD: 1991 to 2004'. *American Journal of Medical Genetics. Part B, Neuropsychiatric Genetics: The Official Publication of the International Society of Psychiatric Genetics*, 132B (1), 109–125.

Bolte, S., S. Knecht and F. Poustka (2007). 'A case-control study of personality style and psychopathology in parents of subjects with autism'. *Journal of Autism and Developmental Disorders*, 37 (2), 243–250.

Boyden, P., M. Muniz and M. Laxton-Kane (2013). 'Listening to the views of children with learning disabilities: an evaluation of a learning disability CAMHS service'. *Journal of Intellectual Disabilities*, 17 (1), 51–63.

Bowlby, J. (1951). *Maternal Care and Mental Health*. Geneva, World Health Organization (WHO).

Bowlby, J. (1969). *Attachment and Loss*. London, The Hogarth Press.

Bowlby, J. (1980). *Attachment and Loss: Loss, Sadness and Depression*. Volume 3. New York, Basic Books.

Bowlby, J., M. Ainsworth, M. Bostom and D. Rosenbluth (1956). 'The effects of mother–child separation: a follow up study'. *British Journal Medical Psychology*, 29, 211–247.

BPS and RCP (2009). *Attention Deficit Hyperactivity Disorder: Diagnosis and Management of ADHD in Children, Young People and Adults*. National Clinical Practice Guideline Number 72. Downloaded from www.nice.org.uk/nicemedia/live/12061/42060/42060.pdf (accessed 2 January 2014).

Braganza, S. F. and P. O. Ozuah (2005). 'Fad therapies'. *Paediatrics in Review*, 26, 371–376.

Brazelton, T. B., B. Koslowski and M. Main (1974). 'The origins of reciprocity: the early mother-infant interaction'. In M. Lewis amd L. Rosenblum (eds) *The Effect of the Infant on its Caregiver*. London, Wiley.

British Dyslexia Association (BDA) Information (2012). Downloaded from www.bdadyslexia.org.uk (accessed 2 January 2014).

British Medical Association (BMA) Board of Science (2007). *Fetal Alcohol Spectrum Disorders: A Guide for Healthcare Professionals*. London, BMA.

Bromley, J., D. J. Hare, K. Davison and E. Emerson (2004). 'Mothers supporting children with autistic spectrum disorders: social support, mental health status and satisfaction with services'. *Autism*, 8 (4), 409–423.

Bronfenbrenner, U. (1979). *Ecology of Human Development: Experiments by Nature and Design*. Cambridge, MA, Harvard University Press.

Bronfenbrenner, U. (1989/1992). 'Ecological systems theory'. *Annals of Child Development*, 6, 187–249. In R. Vasta (ed.) *Six Theories of Child Development: Revised Formulations and Current Issues*. London and Philadelphia, Jessica Kingsley Publishers, pp. 133–250.

Bronfenbrenner, U. (1994). 'Ecological models of human development'. In *International Encyclopaedia of Education*, Vol 3, 2nd edn. Reprinted in M. Gauvain and M. Cole (eds) *Readings on the Development of Children*, 2nd edn. New York, Freeman.

Burden, R. and J. Burdett (2005). 'Factors associated with successful learning in pupils with dyslexia: a motivational analysis'. *British Journal of Special Education*, 32 (2), 100–104.

Cadigan, K. and M. Alberts (2009). *Minnesota Family Impact Seminar Briefing Report: Policy Issues in Special Education Finance*. The University of Minnesota's Children, Youth and

Family Consortium (CYFC). Downloaded from www.cyfc.umn.edu/policy/documents/fisreport09.pdf (accessed 22 July 2013).

Carbone, S., A. Fraser, R. Ramburuth and L. Nelms (2004). *Breaking Cycles, Building Futures. Promoting Inclusion of Vulnerable Families in Antenatal and Universal Early Childhood Services: A Report on the First Three Stages of the Project*. Melbourne, Victoria, Victorian Department of Human Services.

Carnelley, K. B., P. R. Pietromonaco and K. Jaffe (1996). 'Attachment, caregiving and relationship functioning in couples: effects of self and partner'. *Personal Relationships*, 3 (3), 257–278.

Carpenter, B. (2000). 'Sustaining the family: meeting the needs of families of children with disabilities'. *British Journal of Special Education*, 27 (3), 135–144.

Children Act (1989). Downloaded from www.legislation.gov.uk/ukpga/1989/41/contents (accessed 6 January 2014).

Children Act (2004). Downloaded from www.legislation.gov.uk/ukpga/2004/31/contents (accessed 16 December 2013).

Children and Families Bill (2013). Part 3. Amended in Public Bill Committee 25.04.13. Bill 168. Downloaded from www.publications.parliament.uk/pa/bills/lbill/2013-2014/0032/14032.pdf (accessed 29 July 2013).

Clarren, S., S. J.Astley, V. M. Gunderson and D. Spellman (1992). 'Cognitive and behavioral deficits in nonhuman primates associated with very early embryonic binge exposures to ethanol'. *Journal of Pediatrics*, 121 (5 Pt 1), 789–796.

Code of Ethics and Conduct (2009). Guidance published by the Ethics Committee of the British Psychological Society. Downloaded from www.bps.org.uk/system/files/documents/code_of_ethics_and_conduct.pdf (accessed 19 December 2013).

Coleman, J. C. and L. Hendry (eds) (1990). *The Nature of Adolescence*. London and New York, Routledge.

Connors, K. (2008). *Connors 3rd Edition ADHD Index*. London, Pearson.

Constantino, J. N. and C. P. Gruber (2005). *Social Responsiveness Scale (SRS)*. Los Angeles, CA, Western Psychological Services.

Cooper, M. and E. Glasper (2001). 'Deliberate self-harm in children: the nurse's therapeutic style'. *British Journal of Nursing*, 10 (1), 34–40.

Cooper, P. (1993). *Effective Schools for Disaffected Students: Integration and Education*. Routledge, London, pp. 47–67, 252–254.

Cope, N., D. Harold, G. Hill, V. Moskvina, J. Stevenson, P. Holmans, M. J. Owen, M. C. O'Donovan and J. Williams (2005). 'Strong evidence that KIAA0319 on chromosome 6p is a susceptibility gene for developmental dyslexia'. *The American Journal of Genetics*, 76 (4), 581–591.

Courchesne, E., C. M. Karns, H. R. Davis, R. Ziccardi, R. A. Carper, Z. D. Tigue, H. J. Chisum, P. Moses, K. Pierce, C. Lord, A. J. Lincoln, S. Pizzo, L. Schreibman, R. Haas, N. A. Akshoomoff and R. Y. Courchesne (2001). Unusual brain growth patterns in early life in patients with autistic disorder: an MRI study. *Neurology*, 57 (2), 235–244.

Cross, M. and A. Vidyarthi (2000). 'Permission to fail'. *Special Children*, 126, 13–15.

Crowell, J. A. and S. S. Feldman (1988). 'Mothers' internal models of relationships and children's behavioural and developmental status: a study of mother–child interaction'. *Child Development*, 59 (5), 1273–1285.

Crowell, J. and S. Feldman (1991). 'Mothers' working models of attachment relationships and mother and child behaviour during separation and reunion'. *Developmental Psychology*, 27 (4), 597–605.

Daily Mail (9 March 2011). Downloaded from www.dailymail.co.uk/news/article-1364321/Michael-Gove-education-reform-cuts-170k-chilldren-special-needs-register.html (accessed 5 January 2014).

Daniel, S. S., A. K. Walsh, D. B.Goldston, E. M.Arnold, B. A. Reboussin and F. Wood (2006). 'Suicidality, school dropout and reading problems among adolescents'. *Journal of Learning Disabilities*, 39, 507.

DDA (1995). Disability Discrimination Act. Downloaded from www.legislation.gov.uk/ukpga/1995/50/contents (accessed 6 January 2014).

DDA (2005). Disability Discrimination Act. Downloaded from www.legislation.gov.uk/ukpga/2005/13/contents (accessed 6 January 2014).

DeFries, J. V., M. Alarcon and R. K. Olson (1997). 'Genetic aetiologies of reading and spelling deficits: developmental differences'. In C. Hulme and M. Snowling (eds) *Dyslexia: Biology Cognition and Intervention*. London, Whurr Publishers.

Dengate, S. and S. Ruben (2002). 'Controlled trial of cumulative behavioural effects of a common bread preservative'. *Journal of Paediatrics and Child Health*, 38 (4), 373–376.

Department for Children, Schools and Families (DCSF) (2008). The Inclusion Development Programme: Supporting Children with Speech, Language and Communication Needs: Guidance for Practitioners in the Early Years Foundation Stage. Archived but available for download at http://webarchive.nationalarchives.gov.uk/20100202100434/http:/nationalstrategies.standards.dcsf.gov.uk/node/175591 (accessed 2 August 2013).

Department for Education (DfE) (2009). *The Team Around the Child (TAC) and the Lead Professional: A Guide for Managers*. London, DfE.

Department for Education (DfE) (2011). *The Activities and Experiences of 19 Year Olds*. London, DfE.

Department for Education (DfE) (2012a). *Support and Aspiration: A New Approach to Special Educational Needs and Disability. Progress and Next Steps*. London, DfE, p. 87.

Department for Education (DfE) (2012b). *Teachers' Standards Guidance DFD-00066-2011* (revised June 2013). Downloaded from https://www.gov.uk/government/publications/teachers-standards (accessed 19 December 2013).

Department for Education and Schools (DfES) (1994). *Code of Practice for the Identification and Assessment of Children with Special Educational Needs (SEN)*. London, DfES/HMSO.

Department for Education and Schools (DfES) (2002). *Code of Practice for the Identification and Assessment of Children with Special Educational Need (SEN)*. London, DfES.

Department for Education and Schools (DfES) (2007). *Social and Emotional Aspects of Learning (SEAL) Programme in Secondary Schools: National Evaluation*. N. Humphrey, A. Lendrum and M. Wigelsworth (eds), pp. 5–7.

Department for Education and Schools (DfES) (2009). *Common Assessment Framework CAF*. London, UK Government.

Department of Health (DH) (2001). *Valuing People: A New Strategy for Learning Disability for the 21st Century*. CM5086 White Paper. Downloaded from www.archive.official-documents.co.uk/document/cm50/5086/5086.htm (accessed 5 August 2013).

Department of Health (DH) (2004). *National Service Framework for Children, Young People and Maternity Services: Executive Summary*. London, DH.

Department of Health (DH) (2009). *Healthy Child Programme: HCP 0–5*. London, DCSF/DH.

Department of Health (DH) (2012). *School Nurse Fact Sheet: Health and Social Care Professionals*. November. London, DH.

Department of Health (DH) (2013). *Giving all Children a Healthy Start in Life*. 25 March. Downloaded from www.gov.uk/government/policies/giving-all-children-a-healthy-start-in-life (accessed 2 January 2014).

Dolan, A. (2013). 'Father's project'. Email (23.06.2013). Warwick University. Qualitative evaluation of fathers' views of attending the Solihull Approach Parenting Group for Fathers. Data being prepared for publication.

Doman, G. and C. Delacato (1968). 'Doman-Delacato philosophy'. *Human Potential*, 1, 112–116.

Donaldson, M. (1987). *Children's Minds*. London, Fontana Press.

Douglas, H. (2011). 'The Solihull Approach: a whole school approach'. *Journal of Educational Psychotherapy*, 18, 53–58.

Douglas, H. and A. Brennan (2004). 'Containment, reciprocity and behaviour management: preliminary evaluation of a brief early intervention (the Solihull Approach) for families with infants and young children'. *International Journal of Infant Observation*, 7 (1), 89–107.

Douglas, H. and M. Ginty (2001). 'The Solihull Approach: changes in health visiting practice'. *Community Practitioner*, 74 (6), 222–224.

Douglas, H. and M. Rheeston (2009). 'The Solihull Approach: an integrative model across agencies'. In J. Barlow and P. O. Svanberg (eds) *Keeping the Baby in Mind*. London, Routledge.

Dworkin, P. H. (ed.) (2000). 'Preventive health care and anticipatory guidance'. In J. P. Shonkoff and S. J. Meisels (eds) *Handbook of Early Childhood Intervention*. 2nd edition. Cambridge, Cambridge University Press.

Ecker, C., A. Marquand, J. Mourao-Miranda, P. Johnston, E. Daly, M. J. Brammer, S. Maltezos, C. M. Murphy, D. Robertson, S. C. Williams and D. G. Murphy (2010). 'Describing the brain in autism in five dimensions: magnetic resonance imaging-assisted diagnosis of autism spectrum disorder using a multiparameter classification approach'. *The Journal of Neuroscience*, 30 (32), 10612–10623.

Eden, G. F., J. W. Vanmeter, J. Rumsey, J. M. A. Maisog, R. P. Woods and T. A. Zeffiro (1996). 'Abnormal processing of visual motion in dyslexia revealed by functional brain imaging'. *Nature*, 382, 66–69.

Eden, G. F., K. M. Jones, K. Capell, L. Gareau, F. B. Wood and T. A. Zeffiro (2004). 'Neural changes following remediation in adult developmental dyslexia'. *Neuron*, 44 (3), 411–422.

Elder, J., M. Shankar, J. Shuster, D. Theriaque, S. Burns and L. Sherrill (2006). 'The gluten-free, casein-free diet in autism: results of a preliminary double blind clinical trial'. *Journal of Autism and Developmental Disorders*, 36 (3), 413–420.

Epstein, J. (1990). *School and Family connections: theory, research, and implications for integrating sociologies of education and family*. Families in community settings: interdisciplinary perspectives. New York, Haworth, pp. 99–126.

Erickson, C. A., K. A. Stigler, M. R. Corkins, D. J. Posey, J. F. Fitzgerald and C. J. McDougle (2005). 'Gastrointestinal factors in autistic disorder: a critical review'. *Journal of Autism and Developmental Disorders*, 35, 713–727.

Erikson, E. H. (1980/1994). *Identity and the Life Cycle*. New York/London, W.W. Norton & Company.

Evans, R. G. and G. L. Stoddart (1990). 'Producing health, consuming health care'. *Social Science and Medicine*, 31, 1347–1363.

Every Child Matters (2003). London, The Stationery Office.

Evidence (2011). *Oral evidence 22.06.2011. Taken Before the Education Committee Examination of Witnesses N. Amies, L. Bailey, M. Fisher and A. Page*. London, The House of Commons. Downloaded from www.publications.parliament.uk/pa/cm201012/cmselect/cmeduc/1170/11062201.htm (accessed 29 July 2013).

Farone, S. V. and S. A. Khan (2006). 'Candidate gene studies of ADHD'. *Journal of Clinical Psychiatry*, 67 (Suppl 8), 13–20.

Feingold, B. F. (1975). 'Hyperkinesis and learning disabilities linked to artificial food flavors and colours'. *American Journal of Nursing*, 75, 797–803.

Ferreri, C. A. and R. B. Wainwright (1984). *Breakthrough for Dyslexia and Learning Disabilities*. Pompano Beach, FL, Exposition Press of Florida.

Field, L. L., K. Shumansky, J. Ryan, D. Truong, E. Swiergala and B. J. Kaplan (2013). 'Dense-map genome scan for dyslexia supports loci at 4q13, 16p12, 17q22; suggests novel locus at 7q36'. *Genes, Brain and Behavior*, 12, 56–69.

Flutter, J. and J. Rudduck (2004). *Consulting Pupils: What's in it for Schools?* London/New York, Routledge Falmer.

France, A., G. Bendelow and S. Williams (2000). 'A "risky" business: researching the health beliefs of children and young people'. In A. Lewis and G. Lindsay (eds) *Researching Children's Perspectives*. Buckingham, Open University Press, pp. 150–161.

Francks, C. S. P., S. D. Smith, A. J. Richardson, T. S. Scerri, L. R. Cardon, A. J. Marlow, I. L. MacPhie, J. Walter, B. F. Pennington, S. E. Fisher, R. K. Olson, J. C. DeFries, J. F. Stein and A. P. Monaco (2004). 'A 77-kilobase region of chromosome 6p22.2 is associated with dyslexia in families from the United Kingdom and from the United States'. *The American Journal of Human Genetics*, 75, 1046–1058.

Frederickson, N. (2010). 'Bullying or befriending? Children's responses to classmates with special needs'. *British Journal of Special Education*, 37 (1), 4–12.

Freitag, C. M. (2007). 'The genetics of autistic disorders and its clinical relevance: a review of the literature'. *Mol Psychiatry*, Jan 12 (1), 2–22.

Frith, U. (1989). *Autism: Explaining the Enigma*. Blackwell, Oxford.

Frith, U. and E. Hill (2003). 'Introduction'. *Philosophical Transactions of the Royal Society B: Biological Sciences*, 358 (1430), 277–280.

Galaburda, A. M., G. F. Sherman, G. D. Rosen, F. Aboitiz and N. Geschwind (1985). 'Developmental dyslexia: four consecutive patients with cortical anomalies'. *Annals of Neurology*, 18, 222–233.

Galbraith, A. and J. Alexander (2005). 'Literacy, self-esteem and locus of control'. *Support for Learning*, 20 (1), 28–34.

Gathercole, S. E. and T. Packiam Alloway (2006). 'Practitioner review: short-term and working memory impairments in neurodevelopmental disorders: diagnosis and remedial support'. *Journal of Child Psychology and Psychiatry*, 47 (1), 4–15.

Gathercole, S. E., T. Packiam Alloway, C. Willis and A. M. Adams (2006). 'Working memory in children with reading disabilities'. *Journal of Experimental Child Psychology*, 93 (3), 265–281.

Gersch, I. S. (1996). 'Involving children in assessment'. *Educational and Child Psychology*, 13 (2), 31–40.

Gillberg, C. (2003). 'Deficits in attention, motor control and perception: a brief overview'. *Archives of Disease in Childhood*, 88 (10), 904–910.

Glascoe, F. P. (2000). 'Evidence-based approach to developmental and behavioural surveillance using parents' concerns'. *Care, Health and Development*, 26 (2), 137–149.

Golden, G. S. (1984). 'Controversial therapies'. *Pediatric Clinics of North America*, 31, 459–469.

Goleman, D. (1995). *Emotional Intelligence: Why it can Matter More Than IQ for Character, Health and Lifelong Achievement*. New York, Bantam Books.

Goleman, D. (1996). *Emotional Intelligence: Why it can Matter More Than IQ*. London, Bloomsbury Publishing.

Goswami, U. (2004). 'Neuroscience, education and special education'. *British Journal of Special Education*, 31 (4), 175–183.

Gottlieb, M. I. (1989). 'Attention deficit disorders, hyperkinesis, and learning disabilities-controversial therapies'. From selected proceedings of the Fourth International Child Neurology and Developmental Disabilities Congress. In J. H. French, I. Rapin, P. Casaer, M. I. Gottlieb and S. Hare (eds) *Child Neurology and Developmental Disabilities: Selected Proceedings of the Fourth International Child Neurology Congress*. Baltimore/London/Sydney/Toronto, Paul H Brookes Publishing, pp. 251–263.

Grigorenko, E. L., F. B. Wood, M. S. Meyer, L. A. Hart, W. C. Speed, A. Shuster and D. L. Pauls (1997). 'Susceptible loci for distinct components of developmental dyslexia on chromosomes 6 and 15'. *American Journal of Human Genetics*, 60, 27–39.

Hagberg, B., F. Hanefield, A. Percy and O. Skjeldal (2002). 'An update on clinically applicable diagnostic criteria in Rett Syndrome'. Comments to Rett syndrome Clinical Criteria Consensus Panel Satellite to European Paediatric Neurology Society Meeting. Baden Baden, Germany, 11 September 2001. *European Journal of Paediatric Neurology*, 6 (0611), 1–5.

Hall, D. M. B and D. Elliman (2003). *Health for All Children* (4th edn). Oxford, Oxford University Press.

Hall, D. and D. Elliman (eds) (2006). *Health for all Children*. Oxford, Oxford University Press.

Hammersley, M. and A. Traianou (2012). 'Ethics and educational research'. British Educational Research Association online resource. Downloaded from www.bera.ac.uk/resources/ethics-and-educational-research (accessed 19 July 2013).

Hannaford, A. (2013). 'Autism, Inc'. *The Guardian Weekly*, 188 (20), 26–29.

Happé, F., R. Booth, R. Charlton and C. Hughes (2006). 'Executive function deficits in autism spectrum disorders and attention deficit/hyperactivity disorder: examining profiles across domains and ages'. *Brain and Cognition*, 61 (1), 25–39.

Health Visitor Implementation Plan Quarterly Progress Report (July–September 2012). Department of Health (DH). Downloaded from https://www.gov.uk/government/publications/second-health-visitor-implementation-progress-report (accessed 29 July 2013).

Healthy lives, healthy people: our strategy for public health in England (2010). Downloaded from www.dh.gov.uk/en/Publicationsandstatistics/Publications/PublicationsPolicyAndGuidance/DH_121941 (accessed 11 May 2011).

HM Government (2006). Working together to safeguard children: a guide to interagency working to safeguard and promote the welfare of children. Downloaded from www.education.gov.uk/publications/eOrderingDownload/WT2006%20Working_together.pdf (accessed 16 December 2013).

HM Government (2010a) Working together to safeguard children: a guide to interagency working to safeguard and promote the welfare of children. Downloaded from www.education.gov.uk/publications/eOrderingDownload/00305-2010Dom-EN-v3.pdf (accessed 16 December 2013).

HM Government (2010b). *Equality Act 2010 Guidance: Guidance on Matters to be Taken into Account in Determining Questions Relating to the Definition of Disability*. London, Office for Disability Issues, HM Government.

Hudson, J. P. (2010). We were Invited to Participate: Dyslexic Pupils' Perception of Intervention Teaching to Improve Spelling Accuracy. Unpublished thesis, University of Gloucestershire.

Human Rights Act (1998). Downloaded from www.legislation.gov.uk/ukpga/1998/42/ (accessed 16 December 2013).

Humphrey, N. (2002). 'Teacher and pupil ratings of self esteem in developmental dyslexia'. *British Journal of Special Education*, 29 (1), 29–35.

Humphrey, N. (2003). 'Facilitating a positive sense of self in pupils with dyslexia: the role of teachers and peers'. *Support for learning*, 18 (3), 130–136.

Humphrey, N. and P. Mullins (2002). 'Personal constructs and attribution for academic success and failure in dyslexia'. *British Journal of Special Education*, 29 (4), 196–203.

Johnson, R. and Wilson, H. (2012). 'Parents' evaluation of "Understanding Your Child's Behaviour", a parenting group based on the Solihull approach'. *Community Practitioner*, 85 (5), 29–33.

Kadesjö, B. and C. Gillberg (2001). 'The comorbidity of ADHD in the general population of Swedish school-age children'. *Journal of Child Psychology and Psychiatry*, 42, 487–492.

Kanner, L. (1943). 'Autistic disturbances of affective contact'. *Nervous Child*, 2, 217–250.

Klasen, H. and Goodman, R. (2000). 'Parents and GPs at cross purposes over hyperactivity: a qualitative study of possible barriers to treatment'. *British Journal of General Practice*, 50 (452), 199–202.

La Valle, I., L. Payne, J. Gibb and H. Jelicic (2012). *Listening to Children's Views on Health Provision: A Rapid Review of the Evidence*. London, National Children's Bureau.

Lamb, B. (2009). *The Lamb Inquiry: Special Educational Needs and Parental Confidence*. Downloaded from http://dyslexiaaction.org.uk/files/dyslexiaaction/the_lamb_inquiry.pdf (accessed 16 December 2013).

Laming Enquiry (2003). *The Victoria Climbié Inquiry: Report of an Inquiry by Lord Laming* (CM5730). Downloaded from www.official-documents.gov.uk/document/cm57/5730/5730. pdf (accessed 16 December 2013).

Lawrence, D. (1996). *Enhancing Self Esteem in the Classroom*. London, Paul Chapman Publishing.

Lefcourt, H. M. (1982). *Current Trends in Theory and Research*. Hillsdale/New Jersey/London, Lawrence Erlbaum.

Leonard, H., J. Silberstein, R. Falk, I. Houwink-Manville, C. Ellaway, L. S. Raffaele, I. W. Engerström and C. Schanen (2001). 'Occurrence of Rett syndrome in boys'. *Journal of Child Neurology*, 16 (5), 333–338.

Levinson, H. N. (1980). *A Solution to the Riddle of Dyslexia*. New York, Springer.

Lewis, A. and G. Lindsay (eds) (2000). *Researching Children's Perspectives*. Buckingham, Open University Press.

Little, L. (2002). 'Middle-class mothers' perceptions of peer and sibling victimization among children with Asperger syndrome and non-verbal learning disorders'. *Issues in Comprehensive Paediatric Nursing*, 23, 43–57.

Livingstone, M. S., G. D. Rosen, F. W. Drislane and G. M. Galaburda (1991) Physiological and anatomical evidence for a magnocellular defect in developmental dyslexia. Proceedings of the National Academy of Sciences of the United States of America-PNAS. 15 September, 88 (18), 7943–7947. Downloaded from www.ncbi.nlm.nih.gov/pmc/articles/PMC52421/ (accessed 2 July 2013) .

Lord, C., M. Rutter, C. DiLavore and S. Risi (2001). *Autism Diagnostic Observation Schedule (ADOS)*. Los Angeles, CA, Western Psychological Services.

Lord, C., M. Rutter and A. Le Couteur (1994). 'Autism diagnostic interview-revised: a revised version of a diagnostic interview for caregivers of individuals with possible pervasive developmental disorders'. *Journal of Autism and Developmental Disorders*, 24 (5), 659–685.

Love, K. M. and T. B. Murdock (2004). 'Attachment to parents and psychological well-being: an examination of young adult college students in intact families and stepfamilies'. *Journal of Family Psychology*, 18 (4), 6000–6008.

Lowenhoff, C. (2004). 'Practice development: training professionals in primary care to manage emotional and behavioural problems in children'. *Work Based Learning in Primary Care*, 2, 97–101.

Mackie, S., A. P. Shaw, R. Lenroot, R. Pierson, D. K. Greenstein, T. F. Nugent, W. S. Sharp, J. N. Giedd and J. L. Rapoport (2007). 'Cerebellar development and clinical outcome in attention deficit hyperactivity disorder-ADHD'. *The American Journal of Psychiatry*, 164 (4), 647–655.

MacNaughton, G., Smith, K. and Lawrence, H. (2004). *Hearing Young Children's Voices. ACT Children's Strategy. Coonsultation with Children Birth to Eight Years of Age*. Canberra, Department of Education, Youth and Family Services.

Maier, S. and M. Seligman (1976). 'Learned helplessness: theory and evidence'. *Journal of experimental psychology*, 105 (1), 3–46.

Main, M. and J. Solomon (1990). 'Procedures for identifying infants as disorganised/disorientated during the Ainsworth Strange Situation'. In M. Greenberg, D. Cicchetti and E. M. Cummings (eds) *Attachment in the Pre-school Years*. Chicago, University of Chicago Press, pp. 121–160.

Maines, B. and G. Robinson (2001). *B/G-STEEM: A Self Esteem Scale with Locus of Control Items*. London, Lucky Duck Publishing.

Maunders, H., D. Giles and H. Douglas (2007). 'Mothers' perception of community health professional support'. *Community Practitioner*, 80 (4), 24–29.

Melton, G. (1987). 'Children, politics and morality: the ethics of child advocacy'. *Journal of Clinical Child Psychology*, 16 (4), 357–367.

Mikulincer, M., P. R. Shaver and D. Pereg (2003). 'Attachment theory and affect regulation: the dynamics, development, and cognitive consequences of attachment-related strategies'. *Motivation and Emotion*, 27 (2), 77–102.

Miles, T. R. and E. Miles (1999). *Dyslexia a Hundred Years On*. Buckingham, Open University Press.

Milford, R., L. Kleve, J. Lea and R. Greenwood (2006). 'A pilot evaluation study of the Solihull Approach'. *Community Practitioner*, 79, 358–362.

Miller, I. G. and B.E. Hanft (1999). 'Building positive alliances: partnerships with families as the cornerstone of developmental assessment'. *Infants and Young Children*, 11 (1), 49–60.

Millward, C., M. Ferriter, S. J. Calver and G. G. Connell-Jones (2009). *Gluten and Casein-free Diets for Autistic Spectrum Disorder (Review)*. The Cochrane Library. Downloaded from http://onlinelibrary.wiley.com/doi/10.1002/14651858.CD003498.pub3/pdf/abstract (accessed 29 July 2013).

Mishna, F. (2003). 'Learning disabilities and bullying: double jeopardy'. *Journal of Learning Disabilities*, 36 (4), 336–347.

Mitchell, D. (2010). *Education that Fits: Review of International Trends in the Education of Students with Special Educational Needs. Final Report*. Downloaded from www.educationcounts.govt.nz/publications/special_education/education-that-fits-review-of-international-trends-in-the-education-of-students-with-special-educational-needs/executive-summary (accessed 29 July 2013).

Mitterauer, M. and R. Seider (1983). *The European Family: Patriarchy to Partnership from the Middle Ages to the Present*. Oxford, Basil Blackwell.

Moore, T., M. Adams and R. Pratt (2013). 'A service evaluation on the Solihull Approach training and practice'. *Community Practitioner*, 86 (5), 26–27.

Morgan, N. (2005). *Blame my Brain: The Amazing Teenage Brain Revealed*. London, Walker Books.

Morris, C. A. (2010). 'Introduction: Williams Syndrome.' *American Journal Med Genet C Semin Med Genet*, 154C (2), 203–208.

Morris, C. A., J. Loker, G. Ensing and A. D. Stock (1993). 'Supravalvular aortic stenosis cosegregates with a familial 6:7 translocation which disrupts the elastin gene'. *American Journal of Medical Genetics*, 46, 737–744.

Morrow, V. (2001a). 'Using qualitative methods to elicit young people's perspectives on their environments: some ideas for community health initiatives'. *Health Education Research*, 16 (3), 255–268.

Morrow, V. (2001b). 'Young people's explanations and experiences of social exclusions: retrieving Bourdieu's concept of social capital'. *International Journal of Sociology and Social Policy*, 21 (4), 37–63.

Morss, J. (1991). 'After Piaget: rethinking cognitive development'. In J. Morss and T. Linzey (eds) *Growing Up: The Politics of Human Learning*. Auckland, Longman Paul, pp. 1–29.

Munro, E. (2011). *The Munro Review of Child Protection: A Child Centred System*. Crown copyright, UK.

Nadkarni, A., A. Parkin, N. Dogra, D. D. Stretch and P. A. Evans (2000). 'Characteristics of children and adolescents presenting to accident and emergency departments with deliberate selfharm'. *Journal of Accident and Emergency Medicine*, 17, 98–102.

NFER (2011). *Teacher Voice Omnibus: May 2013 Survey – Pupil Behaviour*. Downloaded from https://www.gov.uk/government/publications/teacher-voice-omnibus-may-2013-survey-pupil-behaviour (accessed 29 July 2013).

NHS (2008). *Antenatal Care: CG 62*. Downloaded from http://publications.nice.org.uk/antenatal-care-cg62/guidance (accessed 17 July 2013).

NHS Choices (2011). *Genetic Testing is Ethically Sound*. Downloaded from www.nhs.uk/news/2011/04april/pages/hgc-examines-ethics-genetic-testing.aspx (accessed 28 July 2013).

NICE (2008) Antenatal Care: Routine Care for the Healthy Pregnant Woman. Clinical Guidelines March 2008. Downloaded from www.nice.org.uk/nicemedia/live/11947/40145/40145.pdf (accessed 24 December 2013).

NICE Pathways (2012). Social and Emotional Wellbeing for Children and Young People: Strategy Policy and Commissioning. Downloaded from http://pathways.nice.org.uk/pathways/social-and-emotional-wellbeing-for-children-and-young-people (accessed 23 May 2013).

Nicolson, R. and A. Fawcett (1990). 'Automaticity: a new framework for dyslexia research?' *Cognition*, 35 (2), 159–182.

Nicolson, R. L. and A. Fawcett (2001). 'Developmental dyslexia: the cerebellar deficit hypothesis'. *Trends in Neuroscience*, 24 (1), 508–511.

NMC (2008). *The Code: Standards of Conduct, Performance and Ethics for Nurses and Midwives*. Downloaded from www.nmc-uk.org/Documents/Standards/The-code-A4-20100406.pdf (accessed 7 January 2014).

NMC (2011). *The Prep Handbook*. Downloaded from www.nmc-uk.org/Documents/Standards/NMC_Prep-handbook_2011.pdf (accessed 19 December 2013).

NSW Commission for Children and Young People (2004). Downloaded from www.ccypcg.qld.gov.au/pdf/publications/reports/earlyYears2004/earlyyears_full.pdf (accessed 4 January 2014).

Oberklaid, F. and D. Efron (2005). 'Developmental delay: identification and management'. *Australian Family Physician*, 34 (9), 739–742.

O'Brien, G. (2001). 'Defining learning disability: what place does intelligence testing have now?', *Developmental Medicine and Child Neurology*, 43, 570–573.

O'Brien, G. (2006). 'Young adults with learning disabilities: a study of psychosocial functioning at transition to adult services'. *Developmental Medicine and Child Neurology*, 48 (3), 195–199.

OECD-CERI (2002). *Understanding the Brain: Towards Learning a New Science*. Paris, Organisation for Economic Co-operation and Development-OECD/Centre for Educational Research and Innovation.

Office of National Statistics (2005). *Mental Health of Children and Young People in Great Britain*. London, Palgrave Macmillan.

Ofsted (2010). *The Voice of the Child: Learning Lessons from Serious Case Reviews*. London, the Office for Standards in Education, Children's Services and Skills.

O'Leary, C. (2002). Fetal Alcohol Syndrome: A Literature Review Prepared by Colleen O'Leary. National Alcohol Strategy. Publication 3125. Australia, Commonwealth Department of Health and Ageing.

Ollington, N., V. A. Green, M. F. O'Reilly, G. E. Lancioni and R. Didden (2012). 'Functional analysis of insistence on sameness in an 11 year old boy with Asperger Syndrome'. *Developmental Neurorehabilitation*, 15 (2), 154–159.

Paloyells, Y., M. A. Mehta, J. Kunrsi and P. P. Asherton (2007). 'Functional MRI in ADHD: a systematic literature review'. *Expert Review of Neurotherpeutics*, 7 (10), 1337–1356.

Parracho, H., M. O. Bingham, G. R. Gibson and A. L. McCartney (2005). 'Differences between the gut microflora of children with autistic spectrum disorders and that of healthy children'. *Journal of Medical Microbiology*, 54 (10), 987–991.

Parrish, T. and M. Alberts (2009). *Minnesota Family Impact Seminar Briefing Report: Policy Issues in Special Education Finance*. The University of Minnesota's Children, Youth and Family Consortium. Downloaded from www.cyfc.umn.edu/policy/documents/fisreport09.pdf (accessed 23 June 2013).

Pauc, R. (2005). 'Comorbidity of dyslexia, dyspraxia, attention deficit disorder (ADD), attention deficit hyperactive disorder (ADHD), obsessive compulsive disorder (OCD) and Tourette's syndrome in children: a prospective epidemiological study'. *Clinical Chiropractic*, 8 (4), 189–198.

Pelsser, L. M. J., K. Frankena, J. Toorman, H. F. J. Savelkoul, R. Rodrigues Pereira and J. K. K. Buitelarr (2008). 'A randomised controlled trial into the effects of food on ADHD'. *European Child and Adolescent Psychiatry*, 18 (1), 12–19.

Pennesi, C. M. and L. Klein (2012). *Effectiveness of the Gluten-free, Casein-free diet for Children Diagnosed with Autism Spectrum Disorder Based on Parental Report*. Downloaded from www.sciencedaily.com/releases/2012/02/120229105128.htm (accessed 3 May 2013).

Peterson, C., S. F. Maier and M. E. P. Seligman (1995). *Learned Helplessness: A Theory for the Age of Personal Control*. New York, Oxford University Press.

Peterson, R. L. and B. F. Pennington (2012). 'Developmental dyslexia'. *Lancet*, 379 (9830), 1997–2007.

Piek, J. P. and M. J. Dyck (2004). 'Sensory-motor deficits in children with developmental co-ordination disorder, attention deficit hyperactivity disorder and autistic disorder'. *Human Movement Science*, 23 (3–4), 475–488.

Polanczyk, G., M. S. deLima, B. L. Horta, J. Biederman and L. A. Rohde (2007). 'The worldwide prevalence of ADHD: a systematic review and meta-regression analysis'. *American Journal of Psychiatry*, 164, 942–948.

Putnam, R. D. (2000). *Bowling Alone: The Collapse and Revival of American Community*. New York, Simon and Schuster.

Quist, J. F., C. L. Barr, R. Schachar, W. Roberts, M. Malone, R. Tannock, V. S. Basile, J. Beitchman and J. L. Kennedy (2000). 'Evidence for the serotonin HTR2A receptor gene as a susceptibility factor in attention deficit hyperactivity disorder (ADHD)'. *Molecular Psychiatry*, 5 (5), 537–541.

Rack, J. (1994). 'Dyslexia: the phonological deficit hypothesis'. In R. E. Fawcett and R. Nicolson (eds) *Dyslexia in Children: Multi-disciplinary Perspectives*. London, Harvester Wheatsheaf.

Raine ADHD Study (2010). *Long term outcomes associated with stimulant medication in the treatment of ADHD in Children*. Government of Western Australia, Department of Health. Downloaded from www.health.wa.gov.au/publications/documents/MICADHD_Raine_ADHD_Study_report_022010.pdf (accessed 28 July 2013).

Raja, S. N., R. McGee and W. R. Stanton (1992). 'Perceived attachments to parents and peers and psychological well-being in adolescence'. *Journal of Youth and Adolescence*, 21 (4), 471–485.

Rapin, I. and D. Allen (1983). 'Developmental language disorders: nosologic considerations'. In U. Kirk (ed.) *Neuropsychology of Language, Reading and Spelling*. New York, Academic Press, pp. 155–184.

Raven, J. C. (1998, updated 2003) *Raven's Coloured Progressive Matrices (CPM)*. London, Pearson Education.

Reber, A. S. and E. S. Reber (2001). *The Penguin Dictionary of Psychology* (3rd edn). London, Penguin Books.

Richardson, A. (2002). *Fatty Acids in Dyslexia, Dyspraxia and ADHD: Can Nutrition Help?*' Paper presented at Professional Association for Teachers of Students with Specific Learning Difficulties (PATOSS) Conference, keynote paper, April, London.

Rippon, G., J. Brock, C. Brown and J. Boucher (2007). 'Disordered connectivity in the autistic brain: challenges for the "new psychophysiology"'. *International Journal of Psychophysiology*, 63, 164–172.

Robertson, J. (2000). *Dyslexia and Reading: A Neurological Approach*. London, Whurr.

Rose, J. (2009). *Identifying and Teaching Children and Young People with Dyslexia and Literacy Difficulties*. London, DCSF.

Rotter, J. B. (1954). 'The role of psychological situations in determining the direction of human behaviour'. In M. R. Jones (ed.) *Nebraska Symposium on Motivation*. Lincoln, NE, University of Nebraska Press.

Rotter, J. B. (1966). 'Generalised expectancies for internal versus external control of reinforcement'. *Psychology Monograph*, 80 (2), 1–28.

Rotter, J. B. (1990). 'Internal versus external control of reinforcement: a case history of a variable'. *American Psychologist*, 45, 489–493.

Rutter, M. (1972). *Maternal Deprivation Reassessed*. Harmonsworth, Penguin.

Rutter, M., A. Le Couteur and C. Lord (2003). *Autism Diagnostic Interview, Revised (ADI-R)*. Los Angeles, CA, Western Psychological Services.

Safeguarding Vulnerable Groups Act (2006). Downloaded from www.legislation.gov.uk/ ukpga/2006/47/contents (accessed 16 December 2013).

Salt, T. (2010). *The Salt Review: An independent Review of Teacher Supply for Pupils with Profound and Multiple Learning Difficulties (SLD and PMLD)*. Downloaded from http:// webarchive.nationalarchives.gov.uk/20130401151715/https://www.education.gov.uk/ publications/eOrderingDownload/00195-2010BKT-EN.pdf (accessed 16 December 2013).

Sayal, K. (2006). 'Annotation: pathways to care for children with mental health problems'. *Journal of Child Psychology and Psychiatry*, 47 (7), 649–659.

Sayal, K., R. Goodman and T. Ford (2006). 'Barriers to the identification of children with Attention Deficit/Hyperactivity Disorder'. *The Journal of Child Psychology and Psychiatry*, 47 (7), 744–775.

Schaefer, G. B. and R. E. Lutz (2006). 'Diagnostic yield in the clinical genetic evaluation of Autism Spectrum Disorders'. *Genetic Medicine*, September 8 (9), 549–556.

Schaffer, H. R. and P. E. Emerson (1964). 'The development of social attachments in infancy'. *Monographs of the Society for Research in Child Development*, 29 (3), serial number 94.

Schopler, E., M. E. Van Bourgondien, G. J. Wellman and S. R. Love (2010). *Childhood Autism Rating Scale (CARS)* (2nd edn). Los Angeles, CA, Sage.

Scratchley, M. J. (2003). *Hearing their Voices: The Perceptions of Children and Adults about Learning in Health Education*. Unpublished thesis, University of Waikato, New Zealand.

Seligman, M. (1974). 'Depression and learned helplessness'. In R. J. Friedman and M. Katz (eds) *The Psychology of Depression: Contemporary Theory and Research*. New York/ Toronto/London/Sydney, John Wiley and Sons pp. 83–113.

SENDA (2001). Special Educational Needs and Discrimination Act (SENDA). Downloaded from www.legislation.gov.uk/ukpga/2001/10/contents (accessed 7 January 2014).

Shakespeare, T. (2006). 'The social model of disability'. In L. J. Davis (ed.) *The Disability Studies Reader*. New York, Routledge, pp. 197–204.

Sharma, N. (2003). *Still Missing Out? Ending Poverty and Social Exclusions: Messages to Government from Families with Disabled Children*. London, Barnados.

Skinner, B. F. (1938). *The Behavior of Organisms*. New York, Appleton-Century-Crofts.

Smith, A. B. and N. J. Taylor (2000). 'Children's voices'. In A. B. Smith, N. J. Taylor and M. M. Gollop (eds) *Children's Voices: Research Policy and Practice*. Auckland, Pearson Education New Zealand, p. ix.

Smith, R. A. (1995). *Challenging your Preconceptions: Thinking Critically About Psychology*. Pacific Grove, CA, Brooks/Cole Publishing Company, p. 5.

Snowling, M. (1998). 'Dyslexia as a phonological deficit: evidence and implications'. *Child and Adolescent Mental Health*, 3 (1), 4–11.

Spreen, O. (1988). *Learning Disabled Children Growing Up: A Follow-up into Adulthood*. Oxford, Oxford University Press.

Springer, S. P. and G. Deutsch (1997). *Left Brain, Right Brain: Perspectives from Cognitive Neuroscience*, New York, Worth Publishers.

Staller, J. and S. V. Faraone (2006). 'Attention deficit hyperactivity disorder in girls: epidemiology and management'. *CNS Drugs*, 20 (2), 107–123.

Stanley-Cary, C., N. Rinehart, B. Tonge, O. White and J. Fielding (2011). 'Greater disruption to control of Saccades in Autistic Disorder: evidence for greater cerebella involvement in Autism'. *The Cerebellum*, 10 (1), 70–80.

Stanovich, K. E. (1999). 'Forward'. In R. Sternberg and L. Spear-Sperling (eds) *Perspectives on Learning Disabilities: Biological, Cognitive and Contextual*. Boulder, CO, Westview Press.

Stein, J. (2001). 'The magnocellular theory of developmental dyslexia'. *Dyslexia*, 7 (1), 12–36.

Stephanopoulo, E., S. Coker, M. Greenshields and R. Pratt (2011). 'Health visitor views on consultation using the Solihull Approach: a grounded theory study'. *Community Practitioner*, 84 (7), 26–30.

Stephenson, J. and K. Wheldall (2008). 'Miracles take a little longer: science, commercialisation, cures and the Dore Programme'. *Australasian Journal of Special Education*, 32 (1), 67–82.

Stevens, L. J., T. Kuczek, J. R. Burgess, E. Hurt and L. E. Arnold (2010). 'Dietary sensitivies and ADHD symptoms: thirty-five years of research'. *Clinical Paediatrics*, XX (X), 1–5.

Stevenson, J. L. and K. A. Kellett (2010). 'Can magnetic resonance imaging aid diagnosis of the Autism Spectrum?' *The Journal of Neuroscience*, 30 (50), 16763–16765.

Tager-Flusberg, H. (2007). 'Evaluating the theory of mind hypothesis of autism'. *Current Directions in Psychological Science*, 16, 311–315.

Tajfel, H. and J. C. Turner (1986). The social identity theory of intergroup behaviour. In S. Worchel and W. G. Austin (eds) *Psychology of Intergroup Relations*. Chicago, Nelson-Hall, pp. 7–24.

Temple, C. (1999). *The Brain: An Introduction to the Psychology of the Human Brain and Behaviour*. London, Penguin.

Townley, M. (2002). 'Mental health needs of children and young people. *Nursing Standard*, 16 (30), 38–45.

Tripp, G., S. L. Luk, E. A. Schaughency and R. Singh (1999). 'DSM-IV and ICD-10: a comparison of the correlates of ADHD and hyperkinetic disorder'. *Journal of American Academy of Adolescent Psychiatry*, 38 (2), 156–164.

Tronick, E. Z. (1997). 'Depressed mothers and infants: failure to form dyadic states of consciousness'. In L. Murray and P. J. Cooper (eds) *Postpartum Depression and Child Development*. New York, Guildford Press.

TSO (2012). House of Commons Education Committee (2012–13) Pre-legislative scrutiny: Special Educational Needs. Sixth Report of Sessions 2012–13 Vol III. December 19, 2012.

TSO (2013). Children and Families Bill 2013: Contextual Information and Responses to Pre-Legislative Scrutiny. Presented to Parliament February 2013. Cm 8540.

Tulving, E. (1983). *Elements of Episodic Memory*. Oxford, Clarendon Press.

Turner, J. C. and P. J. Oakes (1989). 'Self-categorisation theory and social influence'. In P. B. Paulus (ed.) *The Psychology of Group Influence*. Hillsdale, NJ, Erlbaum, pp. 233–275.

UNCRC (1989). The United Nations Convention on the Rights of the Child (UNCRC). Downloaded from www.unicef.org/crc/files/Rights_overview.pdf (accessed 15 January 2014).

UNCRC (1995). Concluding observations of the Committee on the Rights of the Child: United Kingdom of Great Britain and Northern Ireland. Downloaded from www.togetherscotland. org.uk/pdfs/uncrc%20-%20uk%20first%20concluding%20observations%201995.pdf (accessed 16 November 2013).

UNESCO (1994). *The Salamanca Statement and Framework for Action on Special Needs Education*. Adopted by the World Conference on Special Needs Education: Access and Quality. Salamanca, Spain, UNESCO. Downloaded from www.csie.org.uk/inclusion/ unesco-salamanca.shtml (accessed 29 July 2013).

United Kingdom Public Health Association (UKPHA) (2009). *Health Visiting Matters: Re-establishing Health Visiting*. Downloaded from www.rcn.org.uk/__data/assets/pdf_ file/0011/288290/health_visiting_matters_final_report.pdf (accessed 15 June 2013).

Vygotsky, L. S. (1962). *Thought and Language*. Cambridge, MA, MIT Press.

Vygotsky, L. S. (1978). *Mind in Society: The Development of Higher Psychological Processes*. Cambridge, MA, Harvard University Press.

Walker, A. M., R. Johnson, C. Banner, J. Delaney, R. Farley, M. Ford, H. Lake and H. Douglas (2008). 'Targeted home visiting intervention: the impact on mother-infant relationships'. *Community Practitioner*, 81, 28–31.

Wallbank, S. and S. Hatton (2011). 'Reducing burnout and stress: the effectiveness of clinical supervision'. *Community Practitioner*, 84 (7), 21–25.

Warnock, M. (1978). The Warnock Report. Special Educational Needs: Report of the Committee of Enquiry into the Education of Handicapped Children and Young People. London, HMSO. Downloaded from www.educationengland.org.uk/documents/warnock/warnock1978.html (accessed 7 January 2014).

Weiner, B. (1979). 'A theory of motivation for some classroom experiences'. *Journal of Educational Psychology*, 71 (1), 3–25.

Whitehead, R. and H. Douglas (2005). Health visitors' experience of using the Solihull Approach. *Community Practitioner*, 78, 20–23.

WHO (2011). *World Health Organization (WHO) and The World Bank: World Report on Disability*. Geneva, WHO. Downloaded from www.who.int/disabilities/world_report/2011 (accessed 18 July 2013).

Williams, J. C., B. G. Barrett-Boyes and J. B. Lowe (1961). 'Supravalvular aortic stenosis'. *Circulation*, 24, 1311–1318.

Williams, J. and L. Ross (2007). 'Consequences of prenatal toxin exposure for mental health in children and adolescents'. *European Child and Adolescent Psychiatry*, 16 (4), 243–253.

Williams, L. and Newell, R. (2012). 'The use of the Solihull Approach with children with complex neurodevelopmental difficulties and sleep problems: a case study'. *British Journal of Learning Disabilities*, 41 (2), 159–166.

Wilson, J. M. G. and G. Jungner (1968). *Principles and Practice of Screening for Disease*. Geneva, WHO, Public Health Papers no. 34.

Wilson, P., F. McQuaige, L. Thompson and A. McConnachie (2008). 'Health visitors' assessments of parent–child relationships: a focus groups study'. *International Journal of Nursing Studies*, 45 (8), 1137–1147.

Wing, L. (1981). 'Asperger's syndrome: a clinical account'. *Psychological Medicine*, 11 (1), 115–29.

Working Together to Safeguard Children. Every Child Matters. Change for Children (2006). Updated 2010, 2013. Downloaded from http://webarchive.nationalarchives.gov.uk/20130401151715/https://www.education.gov.uk/publications/eOrderingDownload/WT2006%20Working_together.pdf (accessed 19 December 2013).

Zeffiro, T. and G. Eden (2000). 'The neural basis of developmental dyslexia'. *Annals of Dyslexia*, 50 (1), 1–30.

Index

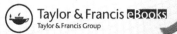